AGELESS MEMORY

AGELESS MEMORY

Simple Secrets for Keeping Your Brain Young

Harry Lorayne

BLACK DOG
& LEVENTHAL
PUBLISHERS
NEW YORK

ISBN-13: 978-1-57912-750-3

Library of Congress Cataloging-in-Publication Data

Lorayne, Harry.
Ageless memory: simple secrets for keeping your brain young/Harry Lorayne.
　p. cm.
Includes bibliographical references and index.
ISBN 978-1-57912-750-3 (alk. paper)
1. Mnemonics. I. Title.

BF385.L737 2008
153.1'2–dc22
　　　　　　　　　　　　2007023981

Book design: Scot Covey

Manufactured in the United States of America

Published by
Black Dog & Leventhal Publishers, Inc.
151 West 19th Street
New York, New York 10011

Distributed by
Workman Publishing Company
225 Varick Street
New York, New York 10014

g f e d c b a

ACKNOWLEDGMENTS

Special thanks to J.P. Leventhal (publisher), Laura Ross (editor), and Jim Mustich. Without them you would not be holding this book right now.

For Renée Lorayne and Robert Lorayne—
what great memories they've given me.

CONTENTS

In the Eye of the "Be Older"

Before I forget…

I've been asked this question many times. I've answered it before. But because this book will be my legacy I'll answer it again— *before I forget*—quickly and succinctly. Oh yes, the question:

How did I, a "dese, dem, and dose" kid from the ghetto of Manhattan's Lower East Side, become "the man with the most phenomenal memory in the world," "the Yoda of memory training" (*Time* magazine, June 2001), the world's foremost memory-training specialist?

It started when I was about eleven years old. Mrs. Goldfisher gave a ten-question test every day. She'd grade each one and we had to take it home so that one parent could sign it. My father (he died when I was twelve) was the "signee," and he punished me just about every school day. Because—I kept getting failing grades, 40s and 50s.

Mrs. Goldfisher said to me more than once, "Harry, you're a seemingly intelligent boy; how come you can't pass these simple tests?" Good question. And it took quite some time before the answer, the "bright light," appeared: a simple, pretty obvious thought that felt to me like an epiphany, an apocalypse, a seminal idea.

The test questions were simple enough. "Who is the vice president of the United States?" I didn't *know*. "What's the capital of Maryland?" I didn't *know*. "What's the main export of Germany?" I didn't *know*. The breakthrough came, the "bright light" danced inside my mind when I realized that I kept saying, thinking, the phrase "I don't know." The word "know" did a few laps around the mental track. Wait a darn minute! Knowing doesn't have as much to do with intelligence as it does with *remembering*. Mrs. G. never asked a test question that hadn't been mentioned or read in class. When I said to myself, "I don't know," I really meant, "I don't *remember.*"

There's no way to intellectualize (I didn't know that word way back then) the capital of a state or the main export of a country. You either know it or you don't. I realized right then that "know," in this context, means the same as "remember." I don't *remember*! (I didn't realize at the time, nor did anyone else since there was no such word, that I was [and am] lysdexic—sorry, I mean dyslexic.)

Oh, my gosh. I realized, if I could learn to remember, I'd get passing grades on these damn tests and, more urgent at the time, my father would stop punishing me. (I once told this story on *The Tonight Show* and included the fact that my father hit me. Negative calls and letters poured into the station. Can't say "hit me." "Punished me" is okay.)

But I obviously had, or thought I had, a lousy memory. (I found out soon enough that there is no such thing.) How can I make myself remember the facts I hear and read in class? In the local library I asked the lady behind the desk (I can still see her in my mind: long black dress, gray hair in a large back-of-the-head bun) if there were any books that teach people how to remember. She directed me to a room way off in an uninhabited corner. I found books on memory training dating back to the seventeenth century. I didn't understand most of what I read; after all, I was only eleven years old. But the tiny fraction I did understand—really, one simple idea—changed my life.

I manipulated that one simple idea so that it worked for me in school, so that it enabled me to remember a fact. And then, when the relevant question appeared on a test, I mentally, joyfully screamed, "I know it! I *know* it!" I had figured out that "know" and "remember" are synonyms; they mean the same thing. If you remember something, you know it; and if you know it—you've *remembered* it. (You've also *learned* it.)

Well, my father stopped "punishing me" and I started to teach that "simple idea" to a few of my classmates. And the years went by. I toyed with that simple idea, enlarged it, twisted and manipulated it so that it "worked" for any kind of information. I became, and am, a motivational speaker. I motivate people to learn how to remember easily and effectively, and to use more, much more, than the proverbial 10 percent of their mental capacities.

I have written many books on the subject, my systems are taught in schools all over the world, and top corporations teach the systems as part of their training programs. I've been written about in literally thousands of magazines and newspapers, and I've written for many of them, too. I've lectured and conducted seminars all over the world: in Australia, Japan, the Philippines, and all over Europe; and I've appeared on major television shows worldwide. In *The Book of Genius* (Stanley Paul Publishers, 1994) there's a paragraph or two talking about a record I set "which may never be broken," that of having met and remembered the names and faces of more than 7,500,000 people during my career, up to that time.

"Time drags you into an alley and beats the _ _ _ _ out of you!" –Mel Brooks

Yes, time does beat the _ _ _ _ out of us, physically and mentally. What's that great, erudite cliché? Oh, yes: growing old sucks! In the movie *All About Eve*, Bette Davis says about growing old, "It ain't for sissies!"

Well, there's another, more recent cliché: "Eighty is the new sixty." (You fill in the ages.)

When it comes to aging, the emphasis, of course, has always been on the physical, and that's probably as it should be. But, I'm here to put *some* emphasis on the mental, particularly for us—and here's that phrase again—"senior citizens." You're going to read this a few times in this book because I can't stress it enough: *It is no longer necessary to accept poor memory, waning memory, loss of memory, or "senior moments" as an inevitable part of growing older!*

With my help, not only will you acquire a memory you never imagined you could have, but you will have it for the rest of your life!

Through the years, I've had many discussions with medical people who have told me that applying my trained-memory systems can hold back senility, even Alzheimer's. Some explained it to me in technical medical terms, how applying my systems sends more blood to and through the brain, and so forth.

Here is some of the medical evidence I've collected that speaks particularly to those of us over 50. And, sorry to disappoint you but this will be the last of any "technical talk." Nothing wrong with "technical talk," of course, but that's not my thing. I'm too results-oriented. I'm interested in giving you a fantastic memory— that's all. But the following quotes are important because they make the point for me.

From *The Journal of the American Medical Association* (2002): "More frequent participation in [mental, mind, brain] stimulating activities is associated with a reduced risk of Alzheimer's."

From *Modern Maturity* magazine: "Just like the heart, the brain needs unclogged arteries to carry fresh blood and oxygen. Help your arteries stay clean by exercising. Any mental exercise *[particularly applying my memory-training systems – HL]* changes the structure of your brain. It causes the nerve cells to grow and the connections between them to strengthen."

A team of researchers led by Dr. Marian Diamond, Professor of Physiology at the University of California at Berkeley reported in *Experimental Neurology* that "even in old age the cells of the cerebral cortex respond to an enriched [stimulating] environment by forging new connections to other cells." Using your mind "increases thickening of the cortex, which is a sign that brain cells *increase in size and activity*. The glial cells (Albert Einstein had an unusually large number) multiply and the grain cells lengthen."

Dr. Diamond's research suggests "that nerve cells grow no matter what one's age, in response to "intellectual enrichment *[read use, exercise; using your imagination and memory]*—anything that stimulates the brain with novelty and change." *And I'm without a doubt going to stimulate your brain with novelty and change!* The research concluded that "development and growth of the brain go on into old age." This fact was noted and repeated in the *New York Times*, June 30, 1985.

From neuropsychologist Marilyn Albert, Ph.D, Harvard Medical School: "Our brains have an innate capacity for change *[and betterment – HL]* no matter how old we are."

From *Aging Myths* (McGraw-Hill) by Dr. Siegfried Kra, Yale University School of Medicine: "Confusion and memory loss are not part of the aging process." I would add to that, "they need not be."

From the *New York Daily News*, (April 30, 1987): "Today's research, including that of the National Institute of Aging, debunks the traditional assumption that aging and forgetfulness go together." *They don't—not necessarily— and I'm here to prove it to you.*

There is absolutely no need for you to continue to complain (or brag) about your terrible memory. No, starting now, you're going to brag about your *terrific* memory!

Enough! Okay, enough about me. The rest of this book is all about YOU! Maybe now your curiosity is piqued and you are ready to discover just how quickly and simply you can learn to regain the memory you had when you were younger—and surpass it— boosting your memory power beyond your wildest dreams.

CHAPTER 1

Pavlov's Dogs

**"My memory is as bad as yours,
my memory is a thousand times better than yours..."**

Read the statement just above again, bearing in mind that I am closer to eighty years of age than I am to seventy. Now let me clarify the remark. As I moved past my forties, the same kinds of memory lapses that annoy and irritate you now annoyed and irritated me. (Don't feel that this makes you "old"—science tells us that our memories start to wane after the age of thirty!) Don't misunderstand. I'm not interested in *only* memory lapses; I'm going to teach you to easily remember *any* new information. But, for the moment, let's focus on those annoying phenomena that some call "senior moments": a name that you've known for years suddenly "escapes" you; someone asks, "What's the word for so and so?" and, though it's a word you've used most of your life, you think for a moment and then say, "You just knocked it out of my mind."

Yes, ordinarily those same "moments" would plague me, too. And my memory, generally, would be as bad, if not worse, than yours. But—and here's the point—when I apply my memory systems, techniques, methods, and tricks, my memory is a thousand times better than yours!

My original working title for this book was a triple header, but my publishers pointed out that it might be a bit unwieldy for a book jacket:

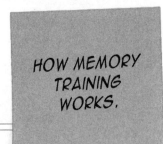

HOW MEMORY
TRAINING
WORKS.

**Where the Hell Did I Put My Keys?!
I Just Had It in My Hands!
Why Am I Staring into the Refrigerator?!**

Sound familiar? Well, not to worry, that's why you're here! Once you've absorbed what's in this book, you'll never have to think like that again. And—call it serendipity or call it of utmost importance—you'll be exercising your mind as you apply my systems. I'm sure you can see why that's important: because exercising the mind isn't all that different from exercising your muscles. It takes a little discipline, it gets harder as you get older, and it is absolutely crucial to staying fit as you age. If you let your arm hang down without using it for a long time, it will eventually atrophy. If you don't exercise your mind, "atrophy" will set in there, too. Even if my systems don't work for you (which, of course, they will, beautifully), you'll be exercising your mind in ways that you never did, or could, before. I've talked and written about exercising your mind for oh so many years. Now, scientific research has caught up with me and has proven that exercising your mind actually builds new brain cells!

That's exciting and important news. It confirms that it's important—no, essential—to exercise your mind. We live in an era of diet and exercise. Everyone is jogging, dieting, running, rowing, bicycling, weight-lifting, treadmilling, ab-building, stair climbing, butt firming, walking, aerobicking, and more. And that's fine. But what good is that great body if you don't have the mental capabilities, the mind power, to go along with it?

There have been and continue to be so many articles written and television shows broadcast wherein "experts" explain the importance of exercising your "cognitive faculties"; your memory and your thinking, decision-making, and problem-solving abilities. They really all send the same message, repeating what I've said for years: *there is no learning and not much thinking without memory.* And these articles and television shows tend to be geared toward the "mature" person. How very important it is, they say, for those of us over forty or fifty years of age to exercise our minds.

Recently, a *New York Times Magazine* section was devoted almost entirely to the research being done on drugs that might help people remember better (if they remember to take them!). Perhaps these "wonder drugs" will be effective and widely available eventually, but it is likely to take many years. And what about those over-the-counter herbs, vitamins, and supplements that claim to improve your memory? Hey, I'm no doctor. Perhaps they can help make your mind a smidgen sharper. There is, however, no way they can give you the kind of memory and mental agility that I can. Perhaps it sounds boastful, but I truly believe that the best memory-enhancing over-the-counter preparation is *me*! (And this book costs a lot less than all of those pills and potions, too.)

Yes, the above-mentioned "news breaks" are always geared toward the older person. (And what the phrase "older person" means is rarely defined, perhaps for good reason. After all, twenty-six is "elderly" to a fifteen-year-old.) I've talked about exercising your mind for years, in response to that frequent complaint, "My memory isn't what it used to be." I call it "the old gray mare" syndrome. Well, let me stress that *it is no longer necessary to accept memory loss as an inevitable consequence of growing older.*

That is just no longer valid.

One of my many unsolicited testimonials came from an eighty-year-old man named Bob Norland. He had had a stroke at seventy-five; his right side was paralyzed and he's now in a wheelchair. He wrote that his doctors told him he'd have tremendous loss of memory. Then, someone brought him one of my books. He went on to say, "Now my memory is much better than it ever was before. It's so good that I give 'memory demonstrations' at my club." Bob does telephone work, he has to return calls—and, because of his stroke, he can no longer write. "But," he says, "I can remember all those names and numbers, and anything else I want to remember, thanks to Harry's memory techniques/tricks. God bless you, Harry."

Intrigued? Read on.

Pavlov's Dogs

Ivan Pavlov, a turn-of-the-century Russian physiologist, psychologist, and physician, was the father of "classic conditioning." In his most famous experiment he proved that, by creating an association in a dog's mind between hearing a bell and receiving food, he could make the dog salivate simply by ringing the bell. It seems like an obvious concept now, but it took Pavlov a bit of time to do his experiment. He continually rang that bell and then immediately gave the dog some food until the dog made the connection between the sound and the reward—until that bell "reminded" the dog of food and made him anticipate it.

You and I are smarter than dogs. We know that, occasionally, if we smell food or simply think about it, we start to salivate. (How about those late-night commercials for pizza and fried chicken? Those advertisers know exactly what they are doing!) We don't need the bell. We can visualize food whenever we want to; we can see it in our mind's eye. Visualizing is part of *thinking*. Aristotle said it three thousand years ago: "In order to think we must speculate with images." Think of something, anything, and you can see an "image" of it in your mind.

What exactly happens in the dog's mind when he hears that bell and is reminded of food? Who knows? Perhaps after many repetitions that sound creates an image of food in the dog's mind. So doesn't it make sense that *we humans* could create a connection in our own minds, so that one thing reminds us of another in the same way? Well, of course we can do that. And, because we can visualize, it is a much faster process than Pavlov used on his dogs—repetition isn't really necessary.

I'll prove that to you. Or better yet, go ahead and prove it to yourself. Isn't there a certain song that, when you hear or think about it, vividly conjures up a specific person, place, or time? I think this has happened to all of us. There may even be a certain smell that starts an avalanche of nostalgia, perhaps sending you back to summer during childhood. One whiff, and you can hear and feel that summer all around you. Hear an old song and the melody *reminds* you of the lyrics, though perhaps you haven't heard or thought about the song in decades.

We are all reminded of different things, people, places, attitudes, ideas, actions, happenings, conversations, and facts many times every day. I bump into an old classmate, we're decades older, and I can "see" that classroom and some of the young people in it. I can see how we all looked at the time, what we wore, what we laughed about. I see it now as I write. I'll wager that you see your own version of it as you read. It's automatic; it's what our mind does for us without being asked; it's part of the human equation. You don't need to take any drugs to make it work! In fact, you can't stop it from working even if you want to—it's a natural phenomenon.

So what in the world does all this have to do with "Where the Hell Did I Put My Keys?" Everything! If a bell can be made to remind a dog of food, why can't your keys be made to remind you of *where they are*?! The answer to that rhetorical question is they can—and they should. And, they can do it without repetition, as I've already told you. You don't need my help when it comes to visualizing—that's a natural phenomenon. What I can do is show you how to harness and corral that phenomenon and use it to your benefit.

Many years ago, the "where-the-heck-is-the-whatever" problem was driving me crazy. Did I solve that particular memory problem (and it *is* a memory problem)? You bet I did. And that solution was the beginning of my quite successful, thank you, career. I call that solution the *Reminder Principle*, but it's really Pavlov's dogs. The "Reminder Principle" is easier for me to talk about, to explain (and even to type!) than "Pavlov's dogs"—so that's it for Pavlov. I'll get a bit deeper into the Reminder Principle in an upcoming chapter, "Absent- to Present-Minded."

As I told you, the memory I was born with is naturally as bad as yours, but it is a thousand times better when I apply my systems. I want you to have the same option. I know of no better way to keep your mind young and keep life exciting, than to create new interests. Creating new interests entails learning new things, amassing new information. You can make your life more interesting right now by learning something exciting and different: namely, my trained-memory methods. Soon, you'll be able to apply those methods to learning lots of other new and different things, easily absorbing new ideas, thoughts, and information.

Please stop thinking that your mental capacity, your memory capabilities, must inevitably decline as you move through "middle age" and beyond. Robert Frost, Georgia O'Keeffe, Pablo Casals, Helen Hayes, Albert Einstein, George Burns, and Carl Sandburg are just a few people who would tell you that it isn't so. They are just a few of the more celebrated examples of people who have done some of their most creative work when they were well into their 70s, 80s, and 90s—and they had highly functional memories and agile minds throughout those "golden years."

Let me stress it again because it warrants repetition: You needn't accept a steep decline in your ability to remember as an inevitable part of growing older!

I know of no better mental exercise than simply to apply, or try to apply, my trained-memory techniques—but I want to break up the process by throwing in a riddle, a puzzle, a "thought provoker"—a mind-power exercise—every so often. I have placed them intermittently throughout the book so you can exercise those brain cells, and you'll come away with some conversation pieces, or ice-breakers, at your fingertips. You'll have fun with them just as you'll have fun, and *enjoy your progress*, with my memory-training systems.

SPECIAL MIND-POWER EXERCISE #1

Add only one symbol to the Roman numeral nine and change it to an even number.

IX

Hint: Drawing a horizontal line through the center of the Roman numeral so that IV shows above that line when you look at it straight on and VI shows above the line when you turn the paper upside down—is not the answer I'm looking for.

Think about it. That, of course, is the point. If you "get it" right away, fine; try it on your friends. If you don't get it right away, keep trying, keep thinking about it. That's the exercise.

All the Mind Exercise solutions are at the back of the book. Don't look at them too soon, though; hang in there—your mental power is certain to surprise you!

CHAPTER 2

Memory Through History

"What goes around comes around."

Quite honestly, if I'd just bought this book instead of having written it, I'd be tempted to skip this chapter! I'd think, "C'mon, get to it, just show me how I can acquire a great memory. That's why I bought the book—not for a history lesson!" But I suggest you take a few minutes to read this chapter. You'll learn just a bit about the history and background of memory training—and a little more knowledge won't clutter your brain, in case you were wondering. You might just find some excellent incentives and enlightening anecdotes here. Of course, you can lick a finger and skip to the next chapter whenever you like, the one that solves and eliminates absentmindedness. But first indulge me for a few minutes.

The Earliest Memory Experts

Memory aids have been used for thousands of years, going back even before ancient Greek and Roman times. Those aids were of utmost importance, particularly to storytellers, orators, and bards. There were no real note-taking devices back then (and even when written language came along, writing materials tended to be cumbersome and impermanent, and few possessed the gift of literacy), so memory aids, systems, and techniques, helped those bards and storytellers remember their songs, poems, stories, and plays.

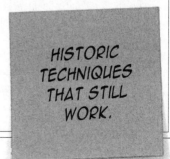

HISTORIC TECHNIQUES THAT STILL WORK.

The orators of ancient Greece and Rome memorized their long speeches thought for thought, by using a technique called *loci*, which means "places." The speaker would mentally connect the first thought of his speech to the first "place" in his home, perhaps the doorway. The second thought was connected with the second place, usually the entryway or foyer, the third idea was connected to the third place, perhaps the stairway, and so on. When he was ready to deliver his speech he'd think of the first place, the doorway, and that reminded him of the first thing he wanted to talk about. When he had completed that thought, he would move on to the second place/thought, and so on, as he took a mental tour through his home. Each place reminded him of a thought and, when he'd completed his mental travels, he'd finished his speech.

From that concept, through the mists of time, developed a figure of speech that we continue to use to this day: "In the first place…, in the second place…, " and so on.

In a four-hundred-year-old Hebrew text (*The Heart of the Lion* by Rabbi Yehuda Aryeh of Medina, published in the year 1611), it is noted that the mandate to use memory systems appears in the Bible as well as in Jewish Talmudic literature. In discussing the importance of learning the Torah, Aryeh quoted the Talmudic scholar Rav Dimi as follows: "One must set signs, schemes/devices, to establish the Torah in those who (try to) learn it. If so, it is enough for us with what has been said by the Bible and our sages (about) Place Memory (loci) and schemes/devices, and their commandment on him to use them."

When the ancient orators, mostly monks and other religious people in those days, felt that their own homes had become too familiar to serve as loci, they wandered the streets searching for other houses, other places to use as memory triggers. In an important step forward, they soon realized that just about anything could be used as loci. The twelve signs of the zodiac, for example, could easily serve as twelve different, sequential places. (Later in this book, I will teach you a quick and easy method for remembering ten to twelve items of any kind, by number, in or out of order. It is a method you can learn in minutes and use for the rest of your life.) Eventually, parts of the Bible were used as "places." What's really interesting is that to use the zodiac signs or parts of the Bible—or anything else—as loci, they first had to learn (remember) those zodiac signs or Bible parts. So the "search" forced them, without their realizing it, to acquire more knowledge!

It was mainly the monks, rabbis, and philosophers of the Middle Ages who were aware of and applied memory-training techniques, and they used them mainly for the purpose of religious teaching. As an example, these systems were used to memorize lists of virtues and vices, and many priests and philosophers taught that using trained-memory systems could show "how to reach Heaven and avoid Hell."

A fragment of parchment dating from approximately 400 BC states, "A great and beautiful invention is memory, always useful for learning and for life." (I was thrilled when I found this in my research because I've written so often that *there is no learning without memory!*) Along similar lines, Aristotle praised memory systems, writing that "these (systems), too, will make a man readier in reasoning." And remember that he also began a book with the statement, "In order to think we must speculate with images." Lovely. Because, again, that's what I do and what I teach: exactly how to *use* mental images. It's a cliché of mine that I will repeat throughout this book: Anything that can be visualized is easier to remember. And anything, I mean ANYTHING, can be visualized—when you know how.

Although Simonides (ca. 500 BC) is considered to be the "father" of the art of trained memory, pieces of parchment dating from over a thousand years before Simonides tell us that memory techniques made up an essential element of the orator's equipment. According to the philosopher Quintilian (ca. 45 AD), "We should never have realized how great is the power of a trained memory, nor how divine it is, but for the fact that it is memory which has brought oratory to its present position of glory."

In *De oratore* ("On the Orator," 55 BC), Cicero described how he applied memory systems and how lawyers and orators of his time were all aided by applying memory systems and techniques. It was known way back then that—and I just love this—memory training would help the *thinking process itself.* I love it because

I've stated that fact so often in my books, lectures, and seminars. Yes, applying my memory techniques will help you acquire a better-than-photographic memory, and it will also give you a much stronger sense of *imagination*, a keener sense of *concentration*, and a much better ability to *observe*, to focus attention. All of these are parts of the thinking process. And those "wheels" of imagination, concentration, and observation automatically and definitely go hand in hand with my trained-memory systems. Those wheels start to spin as rapidly as the "memory wheel" without any extra effort on your part.

In my very first book on the subject, back in 1956, I used an anecdote about speeches at the top of that particular chapter. Here it is, brought up to date a bit:

> *As the nervous speaker approached the microphone his hands went into one pocket after the other, obviously searching for his notes. As he reached the microphone, he murmured haltingly, "My f-f-friends, wh-when I arrived here this evening only G-God and I knew what I was g-g-going to say. N-now only G-God knows!"*

Memory and the Renaissance Man

It's amazing to learn how many powerful people have used memory aids throughout history. Lucius Scipio used them to help him remember the names of *all the people of Rome.* (I've no idea how many people were in Rome then; I'm simply quoting things I learned in my research.) Cyrus (fifth century BC) was able to call every soldier in his army by name. And Seneca (ca. first century AD) could memorize and repeat two thousand words after hearing them once.

Many books on the subject of memory training systems appeared during the fifteenth and sixteenth centuries in Europe. (It was, after all, the Renaissance—a period of great enlightenment when acquiring knowledge was valued above all else.) These, of course, were instrumental in making the general public more aware of the techniques. The best known of these books was *The Phoenix,* written by Peter of Ravenna in 1491. Because of its popularity, many other works on the subject followed. In *The Phoenix,* Peter stated that the best loci are in churches, and by using loci (he is said to have memorized 100,000 places!) he could repeat from memory the entire canon law, 200 of Cicero's speeches and sayings, 20,000 legal points, and more! He offered the example of how he remembers the word *et* by visualizing Eusebius standing in front of Thomas. All he has to do is move Eusebius *behind* Thomas to remember the word *te*. And so on.

The most famous of all Western dramatists, William Shakespeare, had memory aids ("places") built inside of his Globe Theatre to help the actors remember the lines in his plays. The original Globe Theatre, erected in 1599, burned to the ground in 1613 and was immediately rebuilt. Shakespeare, who was a part owner of the building, had a bit to do with its architecture. It was called "the memory theatre" because specific places, or loci, were built into it, places to which the actors might connect the lines, words, and thoughts of a script. Within the theater there were five doors, each of a different color, and five columns, also different colors and shapes, which made up the ten basic loci. The five entrances to the stage were apparently also used as loci, as were the bay windows, entrances, and exits. Other loci included paintings on the ceiling of the zodiac signs and planets, referred to as "the heavens." Very little documented history of the Globe Theatre exists, so much that we know is supposition, based on the documentation of other theaters of the time, but it is fairly certain that Shakespeare himself was a proponent of a sophisticated memory system.

Memory systems were used by King Francis I of France and by England's Henry III. Philosophers of the seventeenth century taught memory techniques; Francis Bacon taught one in his book *The Advancement of Learning.* And some scholars insist that the German philosopher/mathematician Gottfried Leibniz invented calculus as he was searching for a system that would aid in memorizing numbers. (One of my own students memorized pi to the 3,000th place, just to show off!)

One of the most useful things you will learn here is how to visualize ordinarily abstract numbers so that you can memorize them easily, no matter how many digits they contain. And even that is not a new concept. Stanislaus Mink von Wennsshein attempted to do just that in 1648. In 1730, Dr. Richard Grey of England modified the idea. Still, the system was quite clumsy, difficult to apply, and not that helpful. The idea, however, had more than enough merit. I have been told that my simple technique brings the concept to its highest level yet. There now exists an *amazing* technique for memorizing—remembering—numbers.

Memory Training Comes of Age

In a book published in 1888, titled simply *Memory*, philosopher William Stokes talked about the public's interest in the art of memory training:

> *The educated, the intelligent masses, the world, know not and seem not to care to know its (art of memory training) wondrous worth. The adoption of the art by a few paltry thousands cannot be regarded as anything when we consider the countless myriads peopling the earth—when we realize that it is essential to the proper exercise and full development of our intellectual existence as proper breathing is to our physical well-being.*
>
> *There can be little doubt that before long, it will be generally recognized as an established science; and posterity will look back, and regard this plea on behalf of memory as an indication of the intellectual darkness of this age of boasted enlightenment. Let us hope that the day will come when it shall be considered as great a disgrace not to use memory-improvement systems as it is at present not to read!*

Amen. I certainly hope I'm helping to achieve that goal!

I think I've proved (and hopefully not belabored) the point that there's really nothing new about trained-memory systems, memory aids, and the like. What happened, unfortunately, is that the idea of training one's memory fell into disuse for centuries. It's interesting that, in the nineteenth century, some people who did use memory systems publicly were thought to be witches! (If I were around then, I'd have been burned at the stake.) As a matter of fact, the verb "to finagle" is derived from the surname of Gregor von Feinaigle (1760–1819), who wrote a book on memory training a couple of hundred years ago. He was well known in Great Britain for his mental manipulation skills and his number codes. (Another witch, no doubt!)

Like Feinaigle, others started using and demonstrating memory techniques as entertainment. In America during the vaudeville era at the dawn of the twentieth century, performers used memory techniques as a kind of magic act, to amaze audiences with their astonishing mental feats. But the systems were rarely used for practical purposes or serious learning. Occasionally, rarely, someone would attempt to popularize the idea of using trained-memory methods for practical purposes, to increase mental agility in all areas of daily life—but usually without success—until I came along!

Nowadays, many well-known actors use my memory techniques whenever they tackle a new play or movie script. An Academy Award winner, the late Anne Bancroft, wrote to me, "Thank you for making the drudgery [of memorizing scripts] part of my creative art. You are a Miracle Worker!" Alan Alda applies my systems to every script; he talks about it in his book, *Never Have Your Dog Stuffed*, and he has said, "Harry Lorayne can make you remember an address book full of phone numbers as if it were your first kiss. When I go onstage with a hundred pages of text in my head, they got there thanks to the Method: the Harry Lorayne Method."

And it's not just actors. One night, my wife and I had just finished dinner in a popular Long Island restaurant when I was introduced to (then) Secretary of State, Colin Powell. When he heard my name, he threw his arms around me and exclaimed, "Harry Lorayne! You helped make me a general!"

There are many others. And now I hope to expand my efforts even further by concentrating on how my own well-honed systems can be applied to slow, stop, even reverse the mental deterioration that can come with age. You don't have to be slower and duller with each passing year! Take it from me—you can be sharper, clearer, and more mentally agile tomorrow and every day after that. Read on.

SPECIAL MIND-POWER EXERCISE #2

It's really a simple riddle, but you'll get some mental exercise trying to find the answer.

"Forward I'm heavy, backward I'm not. What am I?"

Spend some time thinking about it. You can do that while you're doing a physical exercise, such as walking, jogging, bicycling, or even brushing your teeth.

Keep repeating the riddle to yourself. If you haven't come up with the answer by tonight, turn to the solution.

CHAPTER 3

From Absent- to Present-Minded

"Our thoughts are so fleeting, no device for trapping them should be overlooked." —Henry Hazlitt

Assuming that you have rounded that bend in the road known as "50," do you find yourself suffering from that "I just had it in my hands" malady? Do you sometimes run to your refrigerator, swing open the door, then stare into it wondering what in the world you're there for? Do you waste time searching for your eyeglasses, then find them perched on top of your head? Do you hide treasured items in special places, then forget where they are? Do you continually worry about whether you unplugged the coffeepot, switched off the lights, put on your answering machine, locked the door, and so forth?

Well, you can eliminate absentmindedness simply by being *present*-minded. How? Easy. Think of the action you're doing, or are about to do, *at that moment*; really think about those mundane actions at the moment you execute them. Again, how? Well, let me quote Mr. Hazlitt again: "Our thoughts are so fleeting, no device for trapping them should be overlooked." I call my "device" for achieving present-mindedness "Original Awareness." You need to be aware of an action as it's taking place, not after it has taken place; it's too late then. So I'll give you a "device" for trapping those fleeting thoughts. It's based on what I call the Reminder Principle.

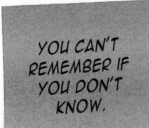

YOU CAN'T REMEMBER IF YOU DON'T KNOW.

I've talked about the phenomenon where songs, smells, and so forth remind us of people, places, ideas, and things. In fact, I doubt that a day goes by without your seeing, hearing, or thinking something that makes you snap your fingers (actually or figuratively) and say, "Oops, that *reminds* me!" What you have seen or heard may have no conscious connection to the thing it reminds you of—but there must be some sort of *sub*conscious connection or one wouldn't have reminded you of the other. And whenever that connection exists, one thing *will* remind you of the other. Again, it's a natural phenomenon.

Now, hear this (I dislike the phrase "listen up"): You can make that kind of a connection *consciously*, knowingly. You can choose what you want to be reminded of, and you can choose the "reminder" itself. Then, not only will that reminder help you figure out where in the world you put your keys or pencil, it will start you along that fascinating road toward having a dependable, reliable, trained memory! And, just as important (if not more so), as you're having fun and amazing yourself with your newfound ability, you are giving your mind the very best possible exercise, building new brain cells just at a time in your life when this is becoming crucial. I'll prove it to you.

Let me ease you into it: I'm writing at my desk. I'm interrupted—the telephone rings, someone calls me with an emergency, or maybe I just need to get a drink of water, and then—"Where the hell is my pencil?" I want to use that same pencil. It takes me fifteen minutes or longer to discover it tucked behind my right ear. Aggravating, annoying, a waste of time. Answering the phone, handling the emergency, getting a drink, those things might only take a couple of minutes, but searching for the pencil can take many times that!

Do I have a solution for that particular problem? You bet I do. And that solution brings us to the Reminder Principle, which is what started all of this memory stuff for me.

Here's an example of the simple idea that will beam you up and away from absentmindedness to a state of present-mindedness. Every time I'm interrupted and I slide my pencil behind my ear, instead of just doing it without thinking, I force myself to see a mental image. I actually see the pencil going *not behind my ear* (that would be too mundane and habitual) but *into* my ear, point first. I can almost feel the pain. I have forced my mind to be "originally aware," to be present *at that instant.* I have trapped a fleeting thought! So later, when I need my pencil, I remember exactly where it is.

Now, because this is the basis of my memory system, because it's so important, I need to take another moment or two to explain it. I need to make you understand that this simple process takes the minutest fraction of the time that it took me to write about it. It's done without breaking mental or physical stride. It's an instant mental calisthenic or exercise.

In that split second, when I formed the mental picture of the pencil in my ear, I brought the Reminder Principle into play, the principle that's always been there, lying dormant. In that split second, I accomplished so much. I forced myself to think of an action that I ordinarily would not think of. I grasped my mind by the scruff of the neck and said, "Darn it, pay attention." I forced myself to think of the action *at that moment.*

The "emergency" is over and I need my pencil again—so I automatically think pencil, no choice. And—"OH, THAT REMINDS ME!"—I can almost feel that pain as my hand automatically moves to my right ear. There's the pencil. No time wasted, no aggravation. Onward.

Have I explained this properly? Reread, please, if you're not sure you understand. This basic idea is the foundation of a system that will enable you to build innumerable "memory steps" for yourself. This principle and its extensions will enable you to remember just about anything—and I don't use the word "anything" lightly. I mean numbers of any kind, from telephone numbers to your Social Security number to your credit card numbers; names and faces; foreign language vocabulary; appointments; errands; thoughts of a speech; reading material—facts of all kinds. Have I whetted your appetite and curiosity? Good. Come along with me. This may be a turning point for you, no matter what your age.

Forgetting to Remember

What does all of this have to do with those questions that crop up more and more as we age, "Where the heck did I put my keys?" or "What did I come in here for?" Everything. Because the method I just discussed using the pencil-in-the-ear example can be applied to anything that you need to keep track of. Let's say you've just unlocked your front door. As you enter, without thinking, you drop your keys into the large flowerpot in your front hall. Of course later, when you are going out again and you need those keys, you complain that you've forgotten where you put them. This is the companion complaint to "I just had it in my hands." (Another favorite is, "I'm introduced to someone and a second later I forget his or her name.")

Please forgive a rusty old platitude of mine, but—you have to *get* something before you can *for*get it. What I'm telling you is that you didn't forget where you put your keys. Nor did you forget his or her name. No...what you did is that you didn't *remember* where you put them in the first place. (You didn't hear and remember that name.) So, you see, you needn't worry that your memory is failing; you haven't applied your memory at all, so you really can't say whether or not it's failing, can you? Seeing that silly picture in my mind (pencil-ear) forced me to think of the action of placing the pencil *at that moment*; it forced me to be originally aware. Information must register in your mind in the first place in order for it to be remembered (or forgotten).

Back to your elusive door keys. From now on and forevermore, you'll never put down your keys without forcing yourself to be "originally aware" of where you're putting them. And rest assured, "forcing yourself" only applies at first; before you know it, you'll simply always do it, not unconsciously, not habitually—that'd defeat the purpose. I want you to put out just a wee bit of effort. But you will do it naturally, without too much trouble.

As you drop your keys into the flowerpot, form a mental image of the two vital entities—the keys and the place where you're putting them. Make it a silly or impossible image. Example: "See" a gigantic key growing in a flowerpot. Perhaps you're watering it to make it grow. It's all one quick picture, thought, or visualization—call it a connection or association—and you've just brought the Reminder Principle into play. Moreover, you've forced yourself to experience original awareness. In that split second, you've registered the action of dropping the keys into the pot in your mind *as it happened*. Your mind was there, present—not absent.

After dinner, you want to go out for the paper and you need to lock the door on your way out. Now, where the hell did you put your keys? Think "key," see a key growing in a flowerpot! Go to that pot in the front hall, retrieve your keys, get on with your life.

Here's another example. Your spouse calls you to come help with something. You put your glasses on the television set as you rush out of the room. When you come back, you spend half an hour searching for the glasses. No more. Now, *as* you put your eyeglasses on the television set (and, again, without breaking mental or physical stride—after all, there may be an emergency to attend to) "see" the TV antenna going through the lens of your eyeglasses, shattering the glass into a million pieces. (Or—"see" a gigantic pair of eyeglasses dancing on television.)

Later, when you're back in the room and you need those eyeglasses, you'll think of them. Needing them means thinking of them, you have no choice. And, if you made that silly mental picture, the Reminder Principle assures that when you think "eyeglasses," you can't help but see them performing on television, or whatever image you have selected. No pause; you walk to the television set, pick up your glasses, and get right back to work. No time wasted, no aggravation, no thinking that your mind is "going." (Or to use another phrase I dislike, that you've had a "senior moment.")

A Reminder Principle connection or association can be made easily, utilizing any two items, even if the second "item" or scenario is abstract and can't ordinarily be seen. I'll solve that problem for you soon enough. I'm stressing any "two" items because most memory problems ultimately break down into entities of two: name to face, foreign word to English equivalent, long number to credit card, name to telephone number, appointment to time or place, and so on.

I've refined the idea, pinpointed it, worried it, made it *work*, but the mental relationship of two items is not a new concept. Socrates, Plato, Aristotle, Saint Augustine, Shakespeare, all understood and utilized it. Saint Augustine referred to it as "coexistence": two ideas active and related in the mind at the same time, no matter how strange or impossible the relationship.

Making the Connection

When you put something in a special place for safekeeping, you can apply the same idea. For example, say you want to save a special pen for your grandchild, so you hide it under a pile of underwear in your top dresser drawer. As you do, form that connection or association between the two things—pen and underwear. Easy enough. "See" lots of ink squirting out of that pen and soaking, ruining, all of your underwear. Each time you think of the special pen, that silly picture will come to mind, until you simply know where that pen is hidden. It becomes *knowledge*.

"Oh, <u>That's</u> What I Came in Here For!"

When my good friend Carl Reiner is onstage and talking about getting older, he says that one of the most common remarks by older people is, "Oh, *that's* what I came in here for!"

"Oops, I need ketchup." The instant you think that thought, "see" gallons of thick, red ketchup pouring all over you. Make the mental picture as silly or impossible as you like—the sillier, the better. I guarantee that you'll know what you came for when you open the refrigerator door—because you've "trapped that fleeting thought" as it tried to "flee" past you!

When you lock your door and you want to remember that you did, see yourself (really *see yourself*) inserting your head or your tongue into the keyhole! Silly? It sure is, but again, you've ordered your mind, forced it, to *pay attention* to this ordinarily habitual, "no thinking required" mundane action. You have forced your mind to be *present* during an action at which it has, for most of your life, been absent. Apply the same idea to help you remember that you've unplugged the coffeepot. As you pull out that plug, see your head, or your spouse's, or a friend's, coming out of the socket. As you push the "on" button of your answering machine, see yourself jumping up and down on that machine to turn it on. It's your call, your choice, your "mind exercise," your solution to an aggravating problem.

You want to be sure to remember to take your umbrella when you leave. If the last thing you see when you leave is, say, the doorknob, "connect" the umbrella to that. Form a silly picture in your mind. Perhaps the doorknob is really a dripping wet umbrella opening and closing, and you are finding it hard to grasp as you try to leave. When you look at that doorknob, you'll know that you have to walk back to get your umbrella. If you always kiss your secretary before you leave the office, you can make *that* remind you of umbrella: See yourself kissing a gigantic wet umbrella. That's all. (Of course, if you walk out into a pouring rain, *that* will certainly act as a reminder!)

Does it all seem silly to you? Good, that's what makes it *work*. And, as it works, it also exercises your mind and strengthens your ability to use your imagination. I'm not interested in a "blue sky" or "pie in the sky" theory. I'm interested in results. I'm nothing if not result oriented.

Silly? I remember a lady asking me to help her to remember that she had a roast in the oven. She said that she's usually reminded of it when she smells it burning. I told her to try putting a small roast in with the regular large roast. Then, when she smelled the small roast burning, that'd remind her that the regular roast was done!

Roasts are too expensive nowadays to use that solution. It's easier, and cheaper, to drop a frying pan or dishtowel or potholder onto the center of the kitchen floor as you put the roast in the oven—anything that's completely out of the ordinary. That will surely keep reminding you of that roast. If you leave the room, say, to watch television, while the roast is cooking, take the frying pan or potholder with you and put it on the floor there, or on the TV set, in full and constant view. You'll have a continual reminder of that roast in the oven!

SPECIAL MIND-POWER EXERCISE #3

A rich Arab dies and leaves his seventeen camels to his three sons. The camels are to be divided as follows:

half to the first son,

one-third to the second son,

and

one-ninth to the third son.

The three sons can't seem to work it out without chopping up some of the camels!

A wise old Arab happens by on his camel and solves the problem immediately—without cutting up any camels.

Do some mental exercise; try to figure out how the wise old Arab did it.

CHAPTER 4

Oh, Pair

If it can be visualized, it is easier to remember.

Some time ago, on a popular national prime-time television show, a segment on memory compared younger people to older ones. One of the tests used by the memory "researchers" was to say the names of ten pairs of items to the subjects. Then the researcher would name one of the items of a pair, out of original order. The subject was supposed to try to name the other item of that pair—the "partner" item.

Good test, I guess. Older people tended to score lower (four or five out of ten) than did the younger people (five or six out of ten). I received hundreds of calls and letters after that segment aired, from people who use my systems, telling me that not only did they "get" all ten items but that they could have done the same with many more pairs. (I later bumped into Hugh Downs, who was the host of that show. I knew him from having met him on *The Tonight Show with Johnny Carson* years before. He told me that NBC had received many calls and letters saying the same thing. Of course, *that* was never aired.)

You can do just as well on the "pairs test," whether you're young, old, or in between, simply by using the one simple idea I've already talked about. Let me prove it to you. Better yet, let me let you prove it to yourself, using just the idea discussed in the preceding chapter.

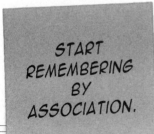

START REMEMBERING BY ASSOCIATION.

Below are ten pairs of items just like those used on the television show. After each one, I've suggested one or more silly "reminder" pictures or associations. Use one of them, or one you think of yourself (that's usually better), and see that picture for just one clear second or so. That's important: see the ridiculous picture and go on to the next one. Laboring over one picture for more than a few seconds defeats the purpose. Do try this. It's important for you to see that it works. (If I said "pencil" to you now that you've read chapter 3, you'd know that the "partner" is ear. If I said "flowerpot," you'd know it is "key.")

BOOK/TREE – You see a million books growing on a tree instead of leaves, or a gigantic book growing like a tree, or a tree reading a gigantic book.

Bear in mind that I want the mental images to be silly, ridiculous, impossible. In this example, seeing a book lying at the foot of a tree is too logical, too mundane, too ordinary. *Those* are the things we tend to "forget" —the everyday mundane things. So make your picture "out of the mundane," make it an impossible, silly picture.

TYPEWRITER/DOG – You're walking a typewriter on a leash instead of a dog, you see the typewriter doing what a dog does when you walk it, or a dog is typing and barking.

LAMP/SCISSORS – You're cutting a lamp in half with a gigantic pair of scissors, or you pull the string on a gigantic pair of scissors and it lights like a lamp.

EYEGLASSES/TV SET – You see the picture I suggested in the previous chapter, or millions of eyeglasses flying out of your TV screen and hitting you in the face; or, you picture yourself wearing a TV set over each eye, instead of eyeglasses.

CAR/DOLLAR BILL – You're driving a gigantic bill instead of a car, or a gigantic bill is driving a car, or you open your car door and millions of dollar bills fly out and cover you.

Are you working along with me? Are you forming (seeing) those silly pictures? Does, for example, "dog" bring the partner item "typewriter" to mind? If not—please—go back and see the ridiculous pictures clearly. If you don't, you're wasting your time. Glance at the pair of words for a moment, form the silly mental picture, then continue.

HAT/BIRD – A hat has wings and is flying, or you're wearing a gigantic flapping bird on your head instead of a hat, or you tip your hat and many birds fly out of it.

TELEPHONE/PEN –You're writing with a ringing telephone instead of with a pen; or you're talking into a gigantic pen instead of into a telephone, perhaps the ink dripping on you as you talk; or a large pen is talking into a telephone.

PICTURE FRAME/PLAYING CARD – You're dealing out picture frames instead of cards and you "see" the glass breaking, or a gigantic card is framed and walks out through the breaking glass.

FISH/BOTTLE – You catch a gigantic bottle instead of a fish, a gigantic bottle is fishing, or bottles are swimming instead of fish.

PAPER CLIP/SINGING – A gigantic paper clip is onstage singing an aria, or millions of paper clips fly into an opera singer's mouth.

If you've managed to "see" a picture for each pair, get ready to surprise and amaze yourself. I'll mention one item of a pair, in no specific order. You fill in the "partner" item. Okay? Try it—what have you got to lose?

PLAYING CARD – Who was playing cards, or what were you dealing out instead of cards? Fill in the "partner" item here: _____ .

LAMP – Think of the image you formed: lamp and _____? You pulled the string and it lit like a lamp. It's _____ .

CAR – You were driving a gigantic _____ instead of a car, or a gigantic one is driving a car, or millions of them fly out of your car.

SINGING – A gigantic _____ is singing. Or millions of them are flying into the face of a singer. It's a _____ .

TREE – Million of them are growing on a tree, or a gigantic one is growing like a tree. It's a _____ .

FISH – You catch a _____ instead of a fish, or a gigantic _____ is fishing.

BIRD – You're wearing a bird instead of a _____ , or many birds fly out of it as you lift it.

TYPEWRITER – A large _____ is typing, or you're walking a typewriter instead of a _____ .

PEN – You're writing with a _____ instead of with a pen, or you're talking into a gigantic pen instead of into a _____ .

EYEGLASSES – You're wearing a _____ over each eye instead of eyeglasses.

How did you do? I'm betting you "got" all or at least nine of them. If you missed one or two, go back and strengthen that picture; that is, see that particular silly picture clearly for a moment, then fill in the following blanks quickly, almost without thinking.

Telephone/ _____	Picture frame/_____
Paper clip/ _____	Dollar bill/ _____
TV set/ _____	Dog/ _____
Scissors/ _____	Fish/_____
Book/ _____	Lamp/ _____
Hat/ _____	Tree/ _____
Singing/_____	Playing card/ _____
Bottle/_____	Typewriter/ _____
Pen/ _____	Bird/ _____
Eyeglasses/ _____	Car/ _____

Are you happy? You should be.

I'm sure you noticed that there were a few words I used quite often as I suggested silly or ridiculous mental images. I used "gigantic" or "millions" and "instead of" in most every case. These words—the exaggeration that they suggest—help you to form ridiculous or impossible mind pictures easily. "Gigantic" will help you see an item much larger than life; "millions" get you to exaggerate the number, the volume, of the item; "instead of" helps you substitute the action of one for the other. (Example: Walking a typewriter on a leash *instead of* a dog.)

Here's my plan. I want you to exercise your mind and, at the same time, acquire a better than photographic memory. And I want you to have some fun while you're doing both. George Bernard Shaw said that if you make people think they're thinking, they'll love you—but if you really make them think, they'll hate you! I don't want you to hate or even dislike me (I thrive on love!) so I'm going to make you really think *without* pain, almost without realizing that you *are* really thinking. Repeat: I want you to have fun while you're thinking!

SPECIAL MIND-POWER EXERCISE #4

A house painter has to paint numbers on the doorway of each of one hundred houses. The numbers are to be consecutive from 1 to 100.

The question is, exactly how many 6s will he have painted when he's completed the job?

Work mentally, not on paper. Counting on your fingers is okay.

39

CHAPTER 5

The Link System

"It is the mundane, ordinary, everyday things that we tend to forget. The unique, the impossible, the ridiculous, the absurd are unforgettable."

You've learned that you can mentally connect or associate any two items so that one will remind you of the other. And that's good; it's really the basis of all trained memory. But let's take it just one small step at a time, starting with my Link System of memory. You will use the Link System to remember things in sequence. You may not realize it, but many things you need or want to remember are sequential: thoughts of a speech, things you read, daily appointments, shopping lists, long numbers, to name just a few of those things.

And, you already know the basic ingredient of the Link System because you learned it in the "Oh, Pair" chapter. That basic ingredient is the ability to *consciously* connect one thing to another. Let's use that ability now. Assume that, for whatever reason, you want to remember the following eight items:

Envelope

Airplane

Wristwatch

Pill

Insect

Wallet

Bathtub

Shoe

Now, as I've told you, you're better off "thinking up" your own ridiculous or

CONTROLLING WHERE YOUR THOUGHTS LEAD.

impossible pictures. When I'm *teaching* the idea, however, I have no choice but to give you examples or suggestions. The reason you're better off creating your own is that then you are *forced* to pay attention to, concentrate on, the two items. My suggestions—my help—may not really be helping you. But if you are aware of that, if you use my suggestion but really *see* that picture in your mind *as if you'd thought of it yourself*, then that's all right.

Okay, back to my list, starting with **Envelope/Airplane**. Begin by visualizing an envelope. Then mentally "attach" that to airplane: a gigantic envelope is flying like an airplane; an airplane is licking and sealing a gigantic envelope; millions of envelopes are boarding or disembarking an airplane; you're trying to stuff an airplane into an envelope. You need only one picture, so select one I've just suggested, or one you've thought of yourself, and *see* it. This has paired *envelope* to *airplane*.

We've made an assumption here. A simple rule of memory is that, to remember something new, it must be connected or associated with something we already know and remember. The assumption we've made is that you "already know" *envelope*. So, we associate the new thing, *airplane*, with that. Let's continue to do that. You now "already know" airplane. So…

Airplane/Wristwatch. The new thing, *wristwatch*, must be brought to mind by airplane. Can you see yourself wearing a large airplane on your wrist instead of a watch? Or maybe there is a gigantic wristwatch around each wing of an airplane, or a gigantic wristwatch is flying like an airplane. I could give you more suggestions, but I'd rather do less than more. *See* one of those pictures in your mind.

Wristwatch/Pill. Think of a silly or impossible picture that features these two items. Did you think of swallowing a watch instead of a pill? Good. Perhaps you saw yourself wearing a large pill instead of a watch. (You see, you can use the "instead of" idea either way in order to make the image memorable.) You could picture a gigantic watch taking a pill. Select one image and *see* it now. Please do not just read my suggestions; really *see* one of the pictures.

Ordinarily you'd go straight through a list such as this. But since this is the first time you're doing it, a quick review might be in order, just to be sure you *are* doing it. Can you think of the first item? (I'll make that easy for you soon.) Envelope, right. What does envelope make you think of, remind you of, right now? Of course, perhaps you were trying to stuff an...airplane into an envelope.

Airplane reminds you of...*wristwatch*. Correct. And *wristwatch* makes you think of...*pill*. Good. Let's continue.

Pill/Insect. Hordes of pills instead of insects are buzzing around you. Or you're swallowing a large insect instead of a pill! (Yucch! Bet you'll remember *that* easily.) You could, of course, see an insect taking a pill. Really *see* whichever mental image you've selected.

You need to see your picture for only a second. It's the clarity of the picture, not the length of time, that's vital. *See* the picture clearly, then go on to the next.

Insect/Wallet. You'll start to see that, within this context, it's the *illogical* picture that comes to mind *before* the logical one. Haven't you already thought of opening your wallet to find millions of insects flying out of it stinging your face? (Action or violence in a picture helps make it ridiculous—and memorable.) Or maybe you thought of wallets buzzing around your head like insects? *See* the picture you've decided on.

Wallet/Bathtub. You're pulling a bathtub (water and all) instead of your wallet, out of your pocket or purse. A gigantic wallet is taking a bath, soaping itself, etc. Pick a pic(ture). *See* it in your mind's eye before continuing.

Bathtub/Shoe. An obviously ridiculous image comes to mind right away: you're wearing bathtubs instead of shoes! Good, that's ridiculous enough. A bathtub is walking, wearing shoes; or a million shoes are overflowing a bathtub. Any of these would do. This is the last item in the list, so be sure to see one of these pictures.

Practicing the Link System

I told you that you'd surprise and amaze yourself when you "did" the pairs in "Oh, Pair." Well, prepare to be amazed again. Think of the first item. If you can't, it might be because I haven't yet taught you how to lock in the first item of a sequential list. You probably already know *envelope*, but if not, just think of any one of the items on the list and go *backward* until you get to *envelope*. What does envelope remind you of? You saw a gigantic envelope flying like an…*airplane*.

Think of *airplane*. What was around each wing? Or, you're wearing an airplane instead of a…that's right, a *wristwatch*.

Think of *wristwatch*. You were swallowing one instead of a…*pill*.

Pills were buzzing around you like…*insects*.

A million insects flew out of your…*wallet*.

You pull something wet out of your pocket or purse instead of a wallet. It's a…*bathtub*.

And you were wearing bathtubs instead of…*shoes*.

Did you know them all? If you missed one, it's because you didn't form/see a *clear* picture originally at that point, or you saw my answer before you thought of it. So, look away so that you don't see the answers, think of envelope—and go through all the items. If you still missed one, go back for a moment, make sure your picture is ridiculous or impossible and, more important, *see* it in your mind *clearly*. Then try going over all the items again.

A Variation

I can't foresee any circumstance where you'd have to remember a link or list such as this *backward*, but just to demonstrate what your mind can do (when it knows how), try this: Think of the last item of your list, *shoe*. What silly picture did you make with *shoe*? Of course, you were wearing a *bathtub* on each foot instead of a shoe. *Bathtub* reminds you of…*wallet*, sure. Keep going, and see if you can go all the way to the first item of this particular list. Of course you can.

Every Good Boy Uses Memory Aids

The idea of taking the mundane or ordinary and making it impossible or ridiculous is certainly not a new idea (though I've been accused of refining, updating, and sophisticating that idea). I've already touched on some of the history of the art of memory so I won't go into it again, except to establish this particular point. *Rhetorica ad Herennium*, from over *two thousand* years ago said, in part:

> *When we see in everyday life things that are petty, ordinary, and banal, we generally fail to remember them. But if we see something exceptionally base, dishonorable, unusual, great or ridiculous, that we are likely to remember for a long time…the striking and the novel stay longer in the mind.*

This was a jolt to me when I discovered it because it reiterates the rule I stated at top of this chapter, a concept I'd been using for decades. Let's go back to Mrs. Goldfisher's tests, which I touched on in the preface: I imagined an apple landing on the head of a classmate named Mary. I actually visualized that, and said to myself, "Look! *An apple is* on *Mary land*ing!" How could I ever forget that the capital of Maryland is Annapolis?

I realize that I'm off on a bit of a tangent here, but bear with me and I'll bring it all back to *aiding your true memory*. Although many educators pooh-pooh memory aids, teachers (at least the ones in the know) have used them for decades. Most everyone I have ever asked remembers the lines on the music staff because a teacher in an early grade told them to think of "*Every Good Boy Does Fine*" (EGBDF). And I know that you remember/know how to recognize Italy on a map because you were once told that it's shaped like a boot.

These examples follow my basic rule of connecting a new piece of information to something you already know. You didn't know the shape of Italy but you knew the shape of a boot. Another excellent example of a memory aid was when one of my teachers in an early grade wanted to help us with the spelling of the word *believe*. It was the *i* and *e* positioning that troubled most of us, so she wrote on the blackboard:

That did it, because we all *already knew* how to spell *lie*. Think of "a *pie*ce of *pie*," and you won't misspell "piece" ever again. I've taken this same idea down a longer road, and I'll go deeper into it later in the book. For now, here's the solution to another problem you might have. Do you have trouble differentiating the masculine or feminine with the names Aubrey/Audrey or Frances/Francis? I know that I've had to help many (including myself) solve the problem of the "difference" over the years. *AuBrey – Boy; AuDrey – Doll, Dame.* Franc*E*s – h*E*r, sh*E*; Franc*I*s – h*I*m, h*I*s. The *b* in Aubrey tells you that it's a boy's name. The *d* in Audrey tells you that it's a "doll's" name. Same for Frances/Francis. What a simple idea. Think of it for just a moment and you'll never again be confused as to which is which.

Here are some more of those "problem solvers." Stationery/ stationary: *stationEry = lEtter; stationAry = stAnding* (still). Or, de*s*ert = *s*and, one *n*; de*ss*ert comes after di*nn*er, double *n*. Do you see how one reminds you of the other? And visualizing many HOMES on a *great lake* will help you remember the lakes *H*uron, *O*ntario, *M*ichigan, *E*rie, *S*uperior. When I wanted to know those same Great Lakes in size order, I thought of: *O*n *E*ach *H*ill *M*an *S*tands. I also formed a picture in my mind of Mt. Fujiyama made up of millions of calendars (12 months, 365 days) so that I could always know that the height of Fujiyama is 12,365 feet!

Controlled Train of Thought

Let's get back to my Link System of memory. You know that quite often—perhaps a few times a day—you think of something that reminds you of something else, then that "something else" makes you think of something else, and that makes you think of...it can go on for a while, but it's really a fleeting train of thought. A train of thought over which you don't have much control. I saw a Pedicab today; that is, sort of like a rickshaw, but drawn by a bicycle instead of a person. It made me think of the same kind of thing I rented in Normandy, France, so that my wife, son, and I could explore the town. That made me think of the wonderful dinner we had in that town that evening, when I saw something on the menu that reminded me of a dish my mother used to make, which made me think of something my mother once said to me…and on and on.

I mention this because it is similar, quite similar, to what you've just accomplished with the Link. Again, a natural phenomenon. The difference is that you have *control* when you apply my Link System. You decide what you want to remember, what you want to be reminded of. It is a *controlled train of thought*.

I mentioned "true memory" a few moments ago. That reminds me to tell you that my systems are aids to your true memory—the memory with which we're all born. In the center of that statistical line all are born with the same capacity for remembering. It's how you use it, apply it, trust it, depend on it, which makes the difference. There's a line between true memory and trained memory, and as you use my trained-memory methods, that line will get thinner and thinner.

Be a Showoff

Before you leave this chapter, why not try another Link or two? Make up your own list, then try to memorize the items in sequence using the Link. You just "did" an eight-item Link—I'll bet that if you can do eight, you can do ten; and if you can do ten, you can do fifteen—who knows how far you can go? Sure, it will take longer to Link twenty items than it will to Link twelve, but that would be the case no matter how you tried to memorize that list of items, whether it was the way you've done it all your life (by rote, through repetition) or by using the new method (Link) you've just learned.

Once mastered, the Link can be a great way to show off the fact that, though you may be getting older, your memory is more amazing than ever. You might have a friend call off, say, a dozen items. He writes them down as he says them; if he doesn't, he'll forget them! Then you can call those items back to him, first forward then backward. But if it's show-off stunts you want, just wait—there's much better stuff later in the book.

As I've suggested, practice by making up your own list of items and Linking them. I'll start you off. Apply what you've learned to the following:

Earring

Salami

Sponge

Chicken

Bucket

Hair

Balloon

Star

Coin

Curtain

SPECIAL MIND-POWER EXERCISE #5

Imagine that there is a bare, unlit lightbulb hanging low in a room. Right around the corner is another room from which the lightbulb cannot be seen. You are in that room, in which there also is a board with three switches on it. Only one of those switches is the on/off switch for the around-the-corner lightbulb; the other two switches are dummies.

Here's the problem: You can throw only one switch to the "on" position. Take your time, change your mind as often as you like, move switches to on and off positions. But you must eventually and finally leave only one switch at "on."

Then you walk into the room with the hanging lightbulb and you have to be able to tell, without leaving the room, *which was the real switch*—1, 2, or 3.

Obviously, if the lightbulb is lit, then the switch you left in the "on" position is the real one. The problem no longer exists. But—what if it isn't lit? Therein lies the problem. Can you solve it? It's not a "trick" question; there is a legitimate answer.

CHAPTER 6

20 Percent Interest

"The true art of memory is the art of attention." —Samuel Johnson

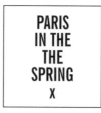

PARIS
IN THE
THE
SPRING
X

Look at the box above. Now look away. What does it say in that box? Did you answer "PARIS IN THE SPRING"? If you did, look again; make sure. I've had people look at it up to seven or eight times and insist that that's what it says: "PARIS IN THE SPRING." Some have read aloud directly from it, looking carefully at it, and still read, "PARIS IN THE SPRING." Then a lightbulb will go off and someone will say, "Oh, I see! It says 'Paris in the spring' with an X at the bottom."

Okay, I don't want to belabor the point. If you haven't spotted it yet, it says "PARIS IN THE SPRING"—plus X. Read it again, pointing to each word with a finger as you do. Oh! Yes, there's an extra "THE" there that few people notice, observe, at first. The X is a small piece of misdirection, it makes the eye travel down that familiar phrase to the X.

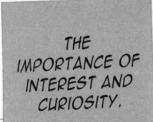

THE IMPORTANCE OF INTEREST AND CURIOSITY.

What I'm talking about here is observation. I wanted to demonstrate that we do not observe as well as we can and should. Observation is a close neighbor of *interest*. It's difficult to separate the two. Before I leave the subject of observation, try something for me. Don't look at your wristwatch, *don't* look at it, and answer this: Is the number 6 on your wristwatch dial the Arabic 6 or is it the Roman numeral VI? Settle on an answer, then check to see if you're correct. Were you? Or, even though you have looked at that watch dial perhaps thousands of times, were you wrong? Or did you just now notice that there *is no* number 6 on your watch dial?!

When I ask this question to a live audience, more than 50 percent of the people are wrong. Then I address those who said they got it right—and if *you* were right I'm addressing you, too—don't look at your watch again. You just did look at it. So…what is the exact time on your watch?

I know, I know, it's a bit of a tricky question, but if I didn't "get you" with that one, I could go on and on until I did "get you." The point is made. There's no way you can remember anything unless you observe it first.

A Matter of Interest

Of course, observation is an important ingredient of memory. How can you remember something if you haven't observed it? Even more important—although, as I've said, it's difficult to separate the two—is *interest*. That is why I titled this chapter "20 Percent Interest"— though I'm sure that the importance of interest in memory is even higher than 20 percent. I'll give you two pertinent examples, one "young" one and the other closer to our age.

This happens so often. A parent brings a child to me, introduces him, and tells me how intelligent he is. He's a smart boy, they say, but he has a terrible memory. He can't remember his schoolwork so he's getting terrible grades. (Many educators insist that a good memory is not important for a student—hah! Just ask a student!)

The boy is twelve years old. He agrees with his mother: he has a terrible memory. I speak to him for only a minute or two, to discover one of his interests. This particular boy is very interested in baseball. Well, as I question him, he overwhelms me with baseball facts: the names and locations of all the teams; the names of all the players, their field positions, batting positions, and which teams they play for; statistics such as runs batted in, home runs, walks, strikeouts, and on and on. Please! A terrible memory? He just proved that he has an *incredible* memory. The important ingredient here is obvious. If that boy could be made to be as *interested* in history, math, science, or any other school subject as he is in baseball, he'd get top grades.

Mr. Bad Memory

Here's another example, geared more to people our age. A man called and said he had "the worst memory in the world." He desperately needed my help. The first thing I told him was that he'd have to get in line behind all the other people who've told me that *they* have the worst memories. (What a great excuse "bad memory" is: "Don't depend on me for anything 'cause I'll forget." The fact of the matter is that every time you say, "I have a bad memory," you put another hole in that sieve of your memory—and give people past fifty a bad name! My goal here is to get you to brag about your *great* memory; and each time you do, you'll plug up one of those holes and tell the world that older can be *better*.)

Back to Mr. Bad Memory. I'll call him Seymour. He went on, "No, no, I'm telling you Mr. Lorayne, I forget to put on my pants in the morning—my memory is that bad. Help!" I was doing a book at the time, so I thought that an interview with Seymour might be a good thing. Seymour and his wife, Molly, were both in the over-fifty group. They ran a mom-and-pop novelty store selling exploding cigars, dribble glasses, whoopee cushions, inexpensive magic tricks. I took Seymour out to dinner; Molly took care of the store.

During dinner Seymour told me more about his terrible memory. I took notes about how he "forgot" to pay the electricity and gas bills and so much more. An hour or so later we walked back to his store. Immediately upon entering, Seymour stopped, started pointing at some merchandise, and said, "Molly, you sold two of those, one of these," and he went on. He knew right away what she had sold during the time we were at dinner!

I said, "Wait just a minute, Seymour; you can tell what's been sold just by looking over the merchandise?" He said, "Well…yeah, usually."

"Let me get this straight; do you know the retail price of each of these hundreds of items?"

"Sure, I have to know that."

"What about their wholesale prices?"

"Yes, of course, I need to know those."

"Their suppliers or manufacturers?"

"Yes."

"What's your biggest selling item?" He pointed it out. "If something was wrong with a shipment of that item, would you know who to call?"

"Sure I would."

"Would you have to look up his telephone number?"

"Oh, no. We do lots of business with him."

"Do you ever forget to pay him, or the bills of any other supplier?"

"Well, no, I can't; I have to pay those bills on time if I want good service."

I looked at him in amazement. "You've spent so much time complaining about your 'worst memory in the world,' yet you remember retail and wholesale prices of hundreds of small items, their suppliers, and the suppliers' telephone numbers. Seems as if you have a damn good memory when something is important to you, when you're *interested*. That's okay; you didn't waste my time. You've given me a chapter for my book!"

I'm sure you get the point: We remember things we're interested in much, *much* better than the things we're not interested in. Pretty obvious, isn't it? And I'm making a fuss about it because I want to bring out the *importance* of the fact that my memory techniques "force" interest and observation *without pain*, without any extra thought or effort. It's *automatic*. That's why this statement, which seems like a contradiction, makes sense: "Even if my systems don't work, they must work."

Of course they work; I've proven that over more than half a century, with literally millions of people. But, even if the systems didn't work, they would definitely bring your memory up to a much higher level. Just *trying* to apply them *forces* you to observe better than you ever have before and *forces* you to be interested, at that moment, in the piece of information you want to remember. As I just took a few paragraphs to prove to you, observation and interest represent a pretty large part of memory in general.

Throw those two things into the "pot" with conscious connections or associations, with the Reminder Principle, with knowing how to visualize anything including abstract information (which I'll be teaching you very soon), and you will be the proud owner of a trained memory, a memory you'll be able to brag about, a memory you never dreamed possible, even when you were twenty-five! Think I'm exaggerating? I'm not. Want to prove it to yourself?

All right, then—onward.

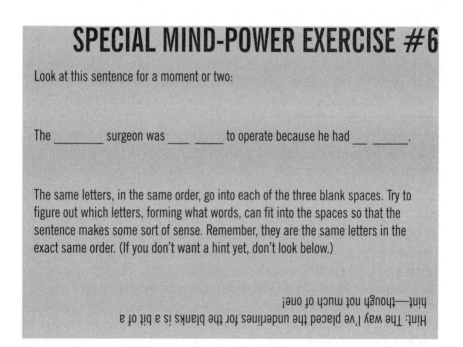

SPECIAL MIND-POWER EXERCISE #6

Look at this sentence for a moment or two:

The _____ surgeon was ___ _____ to operate because he had __ _____.

The same letters, in the same order, go into each of the three blank spaces. Try to figure out which letters, forming what words, can fit into the spaces so that the sentence makes some sort of sense. Remember, they are the same letters in the exact same order. (If you don't want a hint yet, don't look below.)

Hint: The way I've placed the underlines for the blanks is a bit of a hint—though not much of one!

CHAPTER 7

Better, Not Older

"I have discovered the fountain of youth. The secret is simple.
Never let your brain grow inactive and you will keep young forever."
—Georges Clemenceau

Some of my happiest, most appreciative students are people in the fifty-to-over-eighty age group. I receive many testimonials from them, saying, in one way or another, that they want to thank me for giving them something to retire *to* rather than just retiring *from*. (See Bob Norland's testimonial in chapter 1.)

Something interesting to think about: the older you are, the more experience and knowledge you've acquired. The more knowledge you have, the more things you know, so there are more "things" available to you onto which to connect new facts, new pieces of information. So, you see, it's possible that the older you get, the *better* your memory can be! And please forgive my braggadocio, but applying my trained-memory techniques *will definitely* give you a better memory now than you had before, no matter what your age.

I'm sure it's just coincidence, but soon after I decided to do this book I started seeing advertisements and articles about the importance of "jump-starting" your brain. These ads and articles are, of course, directed to the over-forty or over-fifty age group. It turns out that enrollment in adult education courses is booming and the number of applicants in the forty-to-sixty-year-old age range has doubled since 2002. In one New York college alone, these personal fulfillment courses (traditionally in the liberal arts and humanities) have an annual enrollment of more than fifty thousand students. This is good.

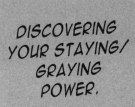

DISCOVERING YOUR STAYING/ GRAYING POWER.

What's not so good are the private courses that offer to "train your brain" in seven to ten lessons, and charge up to $400 for the privilege. From what I can tell, most of them basically give you problems to solve and instruct you to do puzzles, you know, like crossword puzzles. That's something that's mentioned in just about every article I've ever seen that purports to help you exercise your mind: do crossword puzzles. I have nothing against crossword puzzles but please, enough already. Sure, I do 'em, too. I even complete the Sunday *New York Times* puzzle every so often, and sure, they make you think. But, don't fall into a rut. Just trying to apply the techniques you're learning here is thousands of times better for you, in addition to the fact that you'll be "learning a new thing that will help you learn new things!" If you want to take a course—fantastic! Take a real course, where you'll learn something about art, literature, politics, whatever interests you. (It'll even help you with the crossword puzzle—but the crossword puzzle won't help you with much of anything else.)

Incidentally, I know all of the "scientific" words used in some of these supposed "brain-training" programs, words like "eidetic imagery," "sine waves," "left hemisphere and right hemisphere," "short-term memory and long term memory," and on and on. I know them all—but *I don't use them*; you won't find them in this book, or in any of my books. I leave the fancy terminology to the scientists, researchers, and academics who are wonderfully knowledgeable about scientific research. That's all fine if that's what you're interested in, but none of that research, at least not any of it that I know about, teaches you how to better your memory to a fantastic degree, and how to do it *now*. That's *my* job.

Many years ago, when I started to do my own research—and this anecdote should prove my point—there were quite a few "listening" courses available. They ostensibly taught how to listen properly, and a little bit about how to remember what you heard. I checked out quite a few of them. They ranged in cost from $150 to $500, but no matter how much they cost or how many lessons were involved, they all ended basically the same way. After they were done with all of the great-sounding technical terms, they boiled everything down to *two* pretty common words: *pay attention*.

My attitude was, well fine, pay attention—but how? Tell me, show me, teach me, help me learn, *how* to pay attention! Not one of them did. Well, that, among many other good things, is what I do. I teach you how to pay attention. That's *my* job.

Gray Power

In one of my books I included a chapter titled "Staying/Graying Power," geared toward people with gray hair, like me. I included interviews with top executives. Here's an excerpt, a part of my interview with Arlie Lazarus who, at the time, was president and COO (chief operating officer) of Jamesway Corp, which operated over a hundred miniature department stores.

> **Arlie Lazarus:** *I'm getting older. What will happen if I lose my memory? You're really nothing without your memory. I wish you'd discuss that—older people, retired people, the slowing-down process.*
>
> **Me:** *Actually, Arlie, I think that maybe the main reason for the general inefficiency I see today is that people who reach age sixty or sixty-five, who have been doing their work for forty years or so, are forced to retire. These people know what they're doing. They're replaced by young people with little or no experience. And experience is memory, isn't it? Remembering past events in your area of expertise? And I've proven that a person at seventy, seventy-five, or older can have a better memory than they had at age forty! All that's necessary is to know how to properly use, how to stimulate, your memory.*

(After the interview, Mr. Lazarus learned my systems and said, "Harry Lorayne's memory systems will be considered *the* reference for memory training in business, and otherwise, for perhaps the next five centuries.")

Mel Brooks agrees: "In many cases, give me one seventy- or seventy-five-year-old with *experience* over three or four new young people." Mel uses my systems. (He and Anne Bancroft applied the systems—I was there to help, if necessary—to remember the Polish lyrics to "Sweet Georgia Brown," which they sang and danced to at the beginning of Mel's movie *To Be or Not to Be*.) He also says, "Harry Lorayne gives you the memory that will enable you to have knowledge at your fingertips—that will multiply your worth, multiply your value. And you'll even remember what I just said!"

Ralph Destino, then the chairman of Cartier, Inc., after telling me about older people managing Cartier stores, said, "You know what's interesting here, Harry? Someone has to say how important memory is to success, that a great memory distinguishes you immediately, makes you *noticeable*. Harvard Business School doesn't say it—*you* are saying it!"

Well, it boils down to this: Don't allow your enthusiasm, your curiosity, your interest to decline as you grow older. If you keep up those "capacities," your memory will be as strong as ever. The youngest older people I know (and forgive me, but I include me) are those whose interest, enthusiasm, and, therefore, curiosity are still there, still sharp.

Why am I telling you this? Simple. Because learning and applying my memory-training systems, the systems and techniques you'll learn here, will not only exercise your powers of imagination, observation, and concentration, it will automatically force those three "musketeers" into action: interest, enthusiasm, and curiosity.

Perhaps it's true that you can't teach old dogs new tricks. That's dogs, not people. I agree with Benjamin Franklin, who wrote, "No one is ever too old to learn." I try to learn something new every day. I sure tried to "learn something new" when I decided to get "involved" with computers when in my seventies. I was interested, enthusiastic to learn, and certainly curious to see what everyone was talking about.

You need to set up some "mental push-ups"; and applying the techniques, the tricks, you're learning here are the best way to do that. The "Special Mind-Power Exercises" that I've placed after each chapter are the small "extra push-ups." I just want to make sure you're exercising your mind properly. I can't help you physically but I sure can help you mentally. Understand this: there's no better way to stay and feel young than to keep your mind active and working.

That's my goal, and it should be yours.

Just Remember...

You have the same memory capacity as do I or any of my students. You simply need to *know how* to use that God-given memory properly. We've already started you toward that goal. This is the only art or skill I know of that you can start to use immediately—it requires no great advance preparation. You've already successfully applied a basic Link, and it's the use, the application, that's the practice. Let's go on now, let's go a bit deeper into that area of knowledge, that area of "know how."

Remember this: GETTING OLDER IS MANDATORY, GETTING BETTER IS OPTIONAL.

SPECIAL MIND-POWER EXERCISE #7

This should give your mind a good workout!

1. Mrs. Johnson has a bagful of oranges. She bumps into a friend and gives that friend exactly half her oranges—*plus half an orange*.

2. Mrs. Johnson meets another friend and gives her exactly half of her remaining oranges—plus half an orange.

3. Mrs. Johnson bumps into one more friend and gives him exactly half of her remaining oranges—plus half an orange.

4. Mrs. Johnson is left with one whole orange, which she eats.

Your goal is to figure out how many oranges Mrs. Johnson had in the bag at the start.

Hint: There is no knife or juice squeezer involved.

CHAPTER 8

Silver Plate

> "Anything intangible, abstract or unintelligible is easy to remember if it is made to be tangible, meaningful, and intelligible."

What could a chapter with this title possibly be about? Here are three brief anecdotes that illustrate the important concept you'll learn here, starting with the mysterious "silver plate."

It was my son's first visit to France; Robert was three years old. We were having breakfast in our hotel room when he said, "Daddy, why are you always talking about a silver plate?" I said, "What?" He replied, "You say 'silver plate' a lot, Daddy. You just said it to that man with the table." He meant the room service waiter who'd brought in our breakfast on a rolling table. "Oh, Bobby, do you mean *s'il vous plaît*?" I had asked the waiter to set the table "*ici, s'il vous plaît*" ("here, please"). "Uh-huh," said Bobby.

From the mouths, and brains, of babes! Bobby was applying a principle of my system without realizing it of course—he did it automatically. *S'il vous plaît*, French for "please," sounded like "silver plate" to three-year-old Bobby. He was able to remember "silver plate" easily because it meant something to him; he could see it in his mind's eye (just as he always remembered Shakespeare's words, "Bubble, bubble, toil and trouble" because he heard it as "Bubble, bubble, toilet trouble"! Dick Cavett once told me that he thought a popular phrase was "I take it for granite" until he was in his teens, and some children still think a prayer instructs to "Lead us not into Penn Station"!).

"Bobby, that means 'please' in French. It's pronounced..." and I explained it briefly.

FOOLPROOF WAYS TO REMEMBER WORDS AND MEANING.

Later, we were on a beach. A man was walking among the sunbathers, selling French crullers. Bobby asked if he could have one. I told him to run and ask how much they cost. I told him that the word for "how much" is *combien*. Bobby had a friend named Ben. Perfect. I told Bobby to see himself combing Ben's hair—*comb Ben*. Close enough. Bobby laughed. So that he'd remember the meaning of the words, I told him to think to himself *how much* hair Ben had. "And do you remember how to say 'please'?" I asked him. He said he did. He ran to the man, looked up at him, and said, "Comb Ben, silver plate?" Bobby ran back to Renée and me and said, "Five franks (francs), Daddy!"

Another time, I was in Portugal. A bilingual friend and I were having lunch. I had a dish of tiny clams that were delicious. He said that I'd better remember what they were called if I wanted to order them again, because they wouldn't understand the word "clams" in that particular neighborhood. The Portuguese word for "clams" is *Amejues*. The *j* forms a very soft *sh* sound.

I certainly intended to order the clams again, so I took a fraction of a second to form a picture in my mind. I visualized a gigantic clam coming out of the sea. It was dripping with seaweed and sand, it was gritty and dirty looking. As it approached me, I looked at it and said, "What *a mess you is*!" I "said" *mess* with that soft *sh* sound—*what a mesh you is*.

There's that connection, that *reminder*. After that, I simply had to think "clam" and I automatically thought "What a mess you is"— *amejues*. That was forty years ago but I still know the Portuguese word for "clams." How can I ever "forget" it? Bear in mind that after a short while I no longer had to think "what a mess you is" when I wanted the Portuguese word for "clams." What I thought was "*amejues*." I no longer needed the means, I'd reached the end—the result, that is. The word had become *knowledge*.

Substitute Words, Substitute Thoughts

"Silver plate," "comb Ben," "what a mess you is" are examples of what I call Substitute Words or Thoughts. Bobby would have had a bit of a problem trying to remember *s'il vous plait*, but his

"Substitute Thought," his sound-alike, *silver plate*, was no problem at all. The same with *comb Ben*.

Let me backtrack a bit and talk about *English* vocabulary. When I was writing about how to remember vocabulary words close to fifty years ago, I selected some uncommon, unfamiliar English words as examples. I haven't thought about some of them in all of the years since then. They're not words that I would use in normal conversation. And yet, just now, as I was working on this chapter, I thought of one of those words, *endocarp*, and I knew immediately that it meant "fruit (such as peach) pit." Sometimes I amaze even myself! I knew it because I had originally visualized myself hitting a fish, a carp, with a gigantic peach pit. I killed the carp. It was the end of the carp: *end o' carp*. I remembered that outlandish image so I remembered the meaning of the word. (Would researchers file this under "short-term" or "long-term" memory, I wonder?) Can you see that silly picture in your mind?

Let's apply the idea to a few more words that might ordinarily be difficult to remember. (The words I use as examples are not important; the idea, the *technique*, is what is important.) Again, we are dealing with entities of two: the goal is to remember the pronunciation of the word *and* the meaning of that word.

Cantankerous means quarrelsome, cross. Visualize a large tin **can** driving a **tank** and making lots of **errors** (crashing into things, etc.). So you end up with **Can tank errors** ("or us," "arrows," "hurrahs," would do instead of "errors," if that's what came to mind; as would *can tank cross* or *can tan cross*). Using my example, the can that's driving a tank makes errors, which makes the can *quarrelsome* and *cross*. Try to see that picture in your mind (see the can being angry). You can do that in a much shorter time than it just took me to write it, or you to read it.

I was once asked by a college student how to remember the word **resupinate** and its meaning, which is to bend backward. I told him how I would remember it. There was a bowl of alphabet soup on the floor behind me. I bent backward all the way until I could read the soup—and then I ate it. **Read soup and ate** as I *bent backward*! Silly? You bet. That's the point; see that ridiculous picture and you'll know the word and its meaning.

Capricious—fickle, changeable, unsteady. My Substitute Phrase or Thought would be **cap riches.** I might visualize a gigantic cap that's full of riches—cash, jewelry, etc. The cap is handing out the riches (or I'm doing it out of the cap) to different people, then taking it back to give to other people, changing my mind, being fickle. See the picture.

Anchorite is another word for hermit. Can you "see" an anchor writing? Good. See the anchor that's writing as a hermit, perhaps with long hair and a beard, sitting all alone—whatever "hermit" brings to *your* mind. See that picture. **Anchor write**—hermit.

Your **omphalos** is your navel, your belly button. I locked this into my mind by "seeing" my **arm fall loose.** The arm fell right into my belly button! See that ridiculous picture.

Your Turn to Be Amazed

You've amazed yourself a bit already, in preceding chapters. Let's see if you can do it again. If you managed to really *see* the silly pictures I suggested—or those you thought of yourself—for each of the unusual words above, it should be easy for you to fill in the blanks below. Write directly on the page or fill them in mentally.

To be **capricious** is to be _____.

Another word for **hermit** is _____.

The **omphalos** is your _____ _____.

A **fruit pit** is an _____.

Resupinate means to ____ _____.

If you're **quarrelsome**, you're _____.

How'd you do? Are you happy? Try these:

The word for **bend backward** is _____.

The **belly button** is the _____.

If you're **cantankerous**, you're _____.

An **anchorite** is a _____.

An **endocarp** is a _____ ___

If you're **fickle, changeable,** you're _____.

I've said this a few times, and I'll do it many times more, because it warrants repetition: if you missed one, go back and see that picture clearly, then fill in those blanks again.

More Practice

Okay, you've got the idea. I want to be sure you've got it, so let's do a few more. Please do "do" them, because whether you've got the idea or not, doing these Substitute Word or Substitute Thought drills are wonderful mental exercise, as are all of the strategies you'll be learning and applying as you go through this book. You're using not only the "wheel" of memory, but the wheels that go along with it: the wheels of imagination, observation, and concentration. You're making those wheels spin faster than they have in years. What a great way to shake off the mental cobwebs that can come with age—but don't have to! So, even if you already know some of the words I use here, which I'm sure you will, "do" the exercises anyway.

A **factotum** is a handyman, an assistant that does all kinds of work. Visualize a handyman (whatever picture that brings to *your* mind, perhaps a person in overalls, holding tools) writing **facts** on a **totem** pole. (**Fact toe ten** would also do.) Whichever image you select, *see* the picture.

To **castigate** is to scold, criticize, punish. The obvious Substitute Thought is to see someone **casting a gate** and being *scolded* for it, punished or criticized.

Saturnine means gloomy. You **sat on** a gigantic number **nine** and you're very sad and gloomy about it; or the nine is *gloomy* because you're sitting on it. Do you see how thinking up a Substitute Word or Thought *forces* you to concentrate on the word for a second or so?

Rapacity is greediness. See yourself rapping (hitting) a miniature city (**rap a city**) and you do it harder and harder because you're *greedy*. A rapper sitting on a large E would also do—**rapper sit E**.

A **sycophant** is a flatterer. A gigantic ant is flattering you so much that you get sick of that ant: **sick of ant.** See that ridiculous picture.

A **peduncle** is a flower stalk. See yourself paying your uncle (**paid uncle**) with a handful of *flower stalks* instead of money.

Litany is a form of prayer. You lit (burned) your knee (**lit a knee**) and you're praying over the flame. (That's right, I don't care *how* silly you get—the sillier, the better.) See that picture.

Fealty means loyalty. You're **feel**ing a gigantic cup of **tea**. You're asked to feel other things, but you won't, because you're *loyal* to the tea.

To **execrate** is to abhor, hate, or detest. You're stuffing millions of **eggs** into *a* **crate** and you hate doing it. You detest the eggs. Get as much action into your picture as you can; you might see the eggs breaking and getting all over you.

Reminiscent is something that makes you think about past events. You're *rammin'* a gigantic *cent* (**rammin' a cent**) and you're reminded of having done the same thing in the past.

If you've worked along with me you've done ten new words, acquired ten new pieces of information. Please be sure you've really "seen" all the impossible pictures in your mind before you attack the little test that follows.

Fill in the blanks:

> **Execrate** means to _____.
>
> A form of prayer is a _____.
>
> A **sycophant** is one who _____.
>
> A **peduncle** is a _____ _____.
>
> A handyman is a _____.

To be **saturnine** is to be _____.

To think of past events is to be _____.

Rapacity is another word for _____.

To **castigate** is to _____.

Fealty means _____.

Again, if you had a bit of a problem with one or two, it simply means that you didn't form a clear mental picture. Go back and do so now.

Congratulations! You've now learned two of the three major memory techniques or strategies! The first one was the Link System, the connecting of one item to the next to form a "chain." The second one was the Substitute Word or Thought that you've just now mastered. The third major strategy is dealing with numbers. Have no fear, we'll get to that soon.

Even <u>More</u> Practice

Here's some more mental exercise for you. I've provided a list of words and their definitions. For each one, you come up with a Substitute Word, Phrase, or Thought, and an association that holds the key to the word's *meaning*. At the end of the list, I've provided some hints...but come up with your own ideas before you look down at mine.

1. **Abeyance** — temporary suspension.
2. **Sambar** — deer with pointed antlers.
3. **Olfactory** — pertaining to the sense of smell.
4. **Colligate** — arrange in order.
5. **Peripheral** — on the edge, surrounding.
6. **Feasible** — workable; doable.
7. **Agglutinate** — thicken.
8. **Meander** — to wander, walk slowly.
9. **Effete** — exhausted, worn out.
10. **Complacent** — smug, self-satisfied.

Some hints...

1. A **bay** full of **ants** or ants baying at the moon.
2. **Sand bar** or a friend named **Sam** in a **bar**.
3. You enter an **old factory** and are overwhelmed by the terrible smell.
4. **Call a gate** or **collar gate**.
5. **Pear for all**, or **pair overall**.
6. **Fees a bull** (or **bell**); **fees able**.
7. **A glue to Nate**, **egg glued then ate**, or **igloo tin ate**.
8. **Me and her**, or **me enter**.
9. **A feat**; **F eat**; **F feet**.
10. **Come place ant, come play cent, come place cent**.

Final Word

Spinoza said it long before I did. He wrote, "The more intelligible a thing is, the more easily it is retained in the memory, and contrariwise the less intelligible it is, the more easily we forget it." It's amazing how this concept applies to so many areas—including numbers. We'll be getting to them soon enough.

SPECIAL MIND-POWER EXERCISE #8

This will give those brain cells a bit of a workout.

The problem you want to solve is this: You're at the water hose. You need *exactly* seven gallons of water for a gardening project. But...

You have only two buckets available: a five-gallon bucket and a three-gallon bucket.

Using *only those two buckets*, how can you measure out exactly seven gallons of water?

CHAPTER 9

Très Facile Vocabulary Power

All your true, normal memory needs for it to work is a little "reminder."

Well now, here's a bit of serendipity (*Sarah dip a tea*; *surrender pity*) for you: as you learned to "handle" (remember, that is) English vocabulary, you were also learning to handle foreign-language vocabulary. I touched on this at the top of the preceding chapter. (Remember "silver plate"?) In this chapter, we'll expand our vocabulary power to encompass foreign words as well as unfamiliar English ones, using many of the same ideas. If part of your retirement plan is to do that traveling you've wanted to do all your life, this chapter should come in particularly handy. You don't have to "memorize" that foreign phrase book you bought—you can learn the important foreign vocabulary words you need quickly, painlessly—and permanently.

Barry Farber was a popular radio show host for years. (He even ran for public office in New York City.) I was on his show quite often. Barry is also a linguist; he's always been interested in learning languages. In his book on the subject, *How to Learn Any Language,* he wrote, "I almost wept when I first encountered Harry Lorayne's system of committing new words in foreign languages to instant memory—no matter how strange, no matter how long. When I say 'wept,' I mean that I actually cried in rage at all the time I'd wasted attempting to use rote memory of foreign language words before I met Harry Lorayne."

Well, I don't want to make you cry, I'd rather make you happy, so I'll let

MOVING ON TO FOREIGN-LANGUAGE VOCABULARY.

you in on the technique. Two strategies come into play here, the Substitute Word/Thought idea and the Reminder Principle.

An English word that you've never heard before (like **resupinate**) is the same to you as an unfamiliar foreign word, just a strange conglomeration of sounds. If I told you that **singhakom** was an English word meaning so-and-so, you'd apply the strategies you learned in the previous chapter, just as you did for, say, **omphalos**. Actually, *singhakom* is the Thai word for the month of August. To learn it myself, I visualized a gigantic comb singing, a **singer comb** (or *sing ha comb*) and then saw a strong **gust** (of wind) blowing it away. There are your two entities: the reminder of the pronunciation (sing ha comb) and the reminder of the meaning (*gust* for Au*gust*). You can get as specific as you like in your mental pictures. For this one you might visualize yourself saying, "**Aw**" as the **gust** blows away the *singer comb*. The choices are yours; use whatever comes to mind. (For starters, though, do try to "see" the pictures I describe in my examples.)

Psalidi (the *p* is pronounced) is the Greek word for *scissors*. See a gigantic pair of scissors passing a lady: **pass a lady.**

The Swedish word for *sock*, as in a pair of socks, is **strumpa**. See your father strumming (**strum pa**) a gigantic sock instead of a guitar.

Another Swedish word—**byxor**—means *trousers*. See a **big sore** on a pair of *pants*. You can see it bleeding, if you like. If you're a pacifist as I am, any kind of violence is ridiculous. So making the "sore" in this example really gory helps to make the picture more ridiculous, more "mind-grabbing."

Slips (pronounced *sleeps*) means *necktie* in Swedish. Someone **sleeps** on your gigantic *necktie*. It's all so obvious, isn't it? And, yes, my luggage was lost once on a trip to Sweden and I had to do some emergency shopping—so I had to learn/know/remember the words above.

And if you want proof that my systems really work, all you need to do is really see the associations/connections, the silly pictures, I suggest. I'll give you a quick test later. You've nothing to lose, but much to gain. I'll test you on some words from the preceding chapter and some words that I'm using as examples here.

What a simple and seemingly obvious idea. If you wanted to remember that the French word for grapefruit is **pamplemousse**, you might visualize many large pimples on a moose (**pimple moose**) and each pimple is really a *grapefruit*! Really see that picture.

The *i* in *pimple* is pronounced like the *a* in "can." But *pimple* will do it for you because true memory will tell you that it's the *a* sound. Part of the point here is that applying my systems forces you to concentrate on the information as you never have before. That's why your true memory tells you the slight differences. This is so in all areas.

The French word for *cork* is **bouchon** (**push on** or **bush on**). So, you can visualize yourself pushing on a gigantic cork, or you're saying "boo" to a gigantic cork because it is shining a light on you; *boo shone*—cork.

I used the Portuguese word for *clams* (**amejues**) earlier. Here are a few more Portuguese words: **Bolsa** means *purse*. See a gigantic purse made of *balsa* wood, or it's full of balsa wood.

Jantar means *dinner* in Portuguese. Can you visualize a friend named *John* (or the slang word for toilet, *john*) eating *tar* (John tar) for *dinner*? Then do so.

The Portuguese word for *skirt* is **saia**. See a gigantic skirt sighing, it's a *sigher*.

Let's do a few Spanish words. **Estrella** (eh-stray-a) means *star*. See a gigantic letter *S* straying up into the sky, among the stars, or it's straying all the way to a star, and you're admiring it: *S* stray ("ah").

The Spanish word for *window* is **ventana**. See a girl named Anna throwing a vent (perhaps an air conditioner) through a window, which shatters into a million pieces; or a *vent* is blowing *Anna* into a room and out the *window*.

Hermano (pronounced air-mahn-o) is Spanish for *brother*. See your *brother* being an *airman.*

A French word that is difficult for Americans to remember or pronounce is the word for *squirrel*, which is **écureuil.** The "euil" is a sort of "oya" sound. Years ago I was on a television show with the (then) well-known French actor, Jean-Pierre Aumont. We were talking about this word. He told me to say it and as I came to the end sound he squeezed in my cheeks with his hand! Your cheeks do have to sink in for you to pronounce it correctly. Anyway, I thought of *egg cure oil* to enable me to remember the pronunciation; it's pretty close to that conglomeration of sound (although the final *l* is not really pronounced). I "saw" a silly picture of a *squirrel* laying an egg—the *egg* runs to some *oil* to *cure* it—*egg cure oil*.

The idea is easily applied to foreign phrases, as I explained for *s'il vous plait.* The French phrase in the title of this chapter, **très facile**, means **very easy.** "Tray fast eel" would remind of the pronunciation. See an eel on a tray moving fast, and it's doing it very easily.

You've got the idea now. *"C'est trop cher"* (say tro share) is what you'd say when you're shopping in France and you're told a price for an item that's much too high. The phrase means "It's too expensive." See if you can "connect" *say throw share* or *sit row chair* to the meaning of the phrase.

What Have You Learned?

Okay then, it's time for some mind exercise. Using what you've learned above, complete the following:

"**Please**" in French is ___ ____ _____.

Amejues means _____ in Portuguese.

An **endocarp** is a ____ ___.

The **omphalos** is your ____ _____.

The Thai word for **August** is _____.

Très facile means ___ _____.

The Portuguese word **saia** means _____.

An **écureuil** is a _____ in French.

Ventana means _____ in Spanish.

The Spanish word for **brother** is _____.

Estrella means ____ in Spanish.

The Greek word **psalidi** means _____.

Purse is _____ in Portuguese.

The French word **pamplemousse** is a _____.

Check your answers by referring to the text above. As usual, if you missed one or two, you still did some good mind exercise, but go back and strengthen your associations. That is, see the picture clearly then try again.

Foreign Feast

If you travel to foreign countries and eat in restaurants, it behooves(!) you to know the native words for different foods. Let's "do" a partial French menu. I'll give you the pronunciation and perhaps a suggestion for a Substitute Word or Thought, then see if you can connect that to the English food, the meaning. For example, **escargots** are *snails*. See a large *S* in a *car go* slowly like a snail: *S car go*.

Citron (sit run) – *lemon*

Pastèque (pass deck) – *watermelon*. Can you visualize watermelons playing cards as one passes the deck to another?

Homard (oh ma) – *lobster*

Poulet (pool, eh; pool A) – *chicken*

Gâteau (gat, or get, toe) – *cake*

Pain (pan) – *bread*

Beurre (bear, bare) – *butter*

Jambon (jam bone) – *ham*

Glace (glass) – *ice cream*

Champignon (champion yawn) – *mushroom*

Canard (can hard) – *duck*

Ail (eye) – *garlic*

Haricot (the final *t* is silent; airy coat) – *beans*

Haricot vert (airy coat, where) – *green beans*

L'eau (low) – *water*

Pomme – *apple*. See yourself *pumm*eling a gigantic apple, or a gigantic apple is *pumm*eling you.

Form your associations, the ridiculous pictures, then have a friend test you, or test yourself.

Some more mind exercise for you, this time a few Italian food words:

Burro – *butter*. You're smearing butter all over a burro, a donkey.

Carpaccio (car patch *E O*) – *thin raw beef*. You're using thin, pounded, raw beef to put a patch on your car. The patches are shaped like an E and an O.

Agnello (Ann yellow) – *lamb*. Ann turns yellow from eating too much lamb. Or a yellow lamb is named Ann.

Vitello (*V tell O*) – *veal*. Picture a large letter *V tell*ing a large letter *O* about a restaurant that serves veal only.

Calamari (collar, or call her, Mary) – *squid. Collar Mary* and force her to eat a gigantic squid. Or point at a gigantic squid and yell, "Call her Mary!"

Pollo – *chicken*. A gigantic chicken plays *polo*.

And now for some Spanish:

Camarón (camera on) – *shrimp*. A *camera on* a gigantic *shrimp*. (There's an oxymoron for you.)

Huevo (wave *O*) – *egg. Wave O* at a gigantic *egg.*

Sandía – *watermelon*. The watermelon is *sandier* than ever.

Pan – *bread*. You're toasting or buttering a pan instead of a slice of bread.

Pepino – *cucumber.* See a cucumber dancing, running, carrying on—and you say, "Peppy, no?"

Manzana – *apple*. A *man's on a* gigantic apple.

Bentavagnia, Pukczyva, Papadopoulos, Carrasquillo—each a mouthful, but they do not belong in this chapter. Why? Because they can't really be called "foreign language vocabulary." They may, in fact, have meaning if you know the language, but they are proper *names.* Do you see how you might use what you've learned in this chapter to remember names—even complicated foreign ones? If you've tried and applied the vocabulary strategy here, and you've seen that it *works*, you're in for a pleasant surprise.

SPECIAL MIND-POWER EXERCISE #9

This is an interesting mind exercise. I've used it as a conversation opener, an ice-breaker, for years. Some people see it pretty quickly, some never see it.

Try to think of a way that four "that"s can be used in an intelligent sentence, a sentence that has meaning.

Wait—I don't want to make it *that* easy—you have to use the word "that" four times *in a row* (that that that that)!

Remember, it has to be a meaningful, intelligent sentence.

CHAPTER 10

What's in a Name?

"That which we call a rose
By any other name would smell as sweet." —William Shakespeare

"...and be harder to remember!" —Harry Lorayne

Before we get started, project yourself back in time just a bit, say, a few hundred thousand years.

Meet the men of the cave clan: Um, Ug, Il, En, Mool, and Ree. The women have names, too—Ba, Na, Sha, Ra, Nila—but the men rarely use them, particularly the ones who have reached the old age of about thirty-five. Instead, they rely on grunts to call their mates, as grunts are easier to remember than names. But a grunt might summon more than one "she," which makes it necessary for the "he" to indicate which woman he wants through more grunting or by punching the other "she"s away.

The similarity of names complicates the problem. In this particular clan there are a Sa, a Nalee, and a Lina among the females and an Em and an Ulm among the males. Not to mention a Lu, a Ze, and a Rim. Life is hard and uncomfortable, and it becomes increasingly difficult to remember the names. The men spend most of their time hunting for food and the skins they need for warmth. It's dangerous work. The women must build shelters, prepare food, and construct clothing—it's no picnic.

IT PAY$ TO REMEMBER NAMES. HERE'S HOW.

Confusion reigns. Ree calls Ba Sa, Sa calls Um Ulm, En and Em never know which of them is being summoned. Mool never grunts any name at all because at his age (twenty-nine) he just can't remember any of them, much less which name belongs to which clan member.

Now, let's jump forward to the Common Era. "Hi there, Mr. Big Ears; nice to see you, Miss Bushy Eyebrows; I haven't seen you for a while, Mr. Crooked Arm!" At a certain point, people start to call one another by their outstanding features—it's a great improvement! Looking at the person automatically reminds you of that person's name. Most names are descriptive, either of the person's features or of his particular skill. (Today, if your name is Carpenter, Cooper, or Hunter, the odds are that your great [to the nth power] grandfather was a carpenter, a barrel maker, or a hunter.)

If there aren't too many people in the village, there isn't much of a remembering-names problem—but as the birth rate rises, the "system" stops working well because, for example, there are now quite a few people with "jutting chins." And when Ms. Bushy Eyebrows marries Mr. Crooked Arm, she and their offspring are also "Crooked Arms," which means that the name no longer describes all of those who use it. Today, Mr. Cooper is unlikely to be a barrel maker. He may not even know that that's what "cooper" means.

Down through the ages, life has gotten easier and more comfortable in every way. Most of us no longer have to hunt for our food, make our own clothing, or build our own shelters. Women are no longer thought of as men's "property." But there's one problem we haven't managed to solve: how to remember the many names of the people we meet. That's where I come in. Now let's come back to the present day, and tackle the "name problem."

You Can't Remember What You Never Knew

I've seen it so often. I'm seated at the head table at a corporate dinner, waiting for the people to arrive and be seated. Then I can start meeting them in order to remember their names for the opening of my talk. As the doors open, I hear all the standard remarks and exclamations: "Hey, good to see you!" "How've you been?" "How're you doin'?" "Been a while," and so forth. But I notice that most people are not making eye contact. Rather, they are staring at other people's left chest areas!

What they're doing is trying desperately to read one another's plastic name tags. Because, although they recognize the faces, they don't know the names. And (aside from the fact that this little move is embarrassingly obvious), the name tags don't do us much good as we get older because—the old eyesight just ain't what it used to be—and we *can't see the names* on the cards!

It is, of course, the universal memory complaint: "I'm introduced to someone and minutes later I've forgotten his or her name." Well, that just isn't so. You haven't forgotten the name—you didn't remember the name in the first place. I'll take it a step back: you probably didn't even *hear* the name in the first place! Information, *any* information, has to register in your mind if it's to be remembered; you need to be *originally aware* of the information. It's another simple and obvious idea. Why in the world would you expect to remember something that you haven't "registered" in the first place?

Tell you what: I'll give you five rules for remembering names. If you really apply these rules, I guarantee that you'll better your memory for names by about 20 percent. Then I'll teach you my system, which will take care of the bulk of the problem, the remaining 80 percent.

Rule 1: Be sure to hear the name. It is not embarrassing to say, "Sorry, I didn't get your name." Remember that a person's name is his or her most prized possession, so making sure you hear it is flattering to him or her. So be sure to hear the name. That's *basic*. The rest of the rules will simply enable you to apply *this* rule.

Rule 2: Try to spell the name. "Oh, is that L-o-r-r-a-i-n-e?" "No; it's L-o-r-a-y-n-e." Try to spell it and you'll be corrected if you're wrong. Do it with Jones or Smith, it doesn't matter, because you're showing an interest as you make sure you've heard the name right in the first place.

Rule 3: Make a remark about the name. If it's a name you've never heard before, say that. If you think it's a strange name, it's all right to say so. "What an unusual name!" Or, "Oh, I went to school with a Clark Carpenter; is he a relative perhaps?" Any remark will do—and again, you're showing an interest.

Rule 4: Use the name during your initial conversation. Only where apropos, of course, you don't want to sound silly, but do use it as you speak. "Why Jim, I never thought of it that way!"

Rule 5: Say the name when you say goodbye. Don't say, "I'll see you later," or, "I'll see you later, my friend"; instead, say, "I'll see you later, Ms. Gordon."

Religiously apply these five simple rules and you will, you absolutely *must* better your memory for names by twenty percent. But, you really don't have to bother—because if you apply the technique I'm about to teach you, or even just *try* to apply it, those five rules will automatically fall into place for you.

Unzip 'Em

The few names I mentioned at the end of the preceding chapter— Bentavagnia, Pukczyva, Papadopoulos, Carrasquillo—fall into the category of "zip" names; they tend to go in one ear and *zip* right out the other without making the *memory* "pit stop." (Society tells us that we won't remember them anyway, so why bother to try?) Of course, if you apply the rules I just gave you (Rule 1 alone would do it), then those names may "meander," rather than *zip,* into and then out of your memory, but they won't stay there—unless we really unzip them.

Here's that pleasant surprise I mentioned. You're going to apply the very same strategy you have already learned and used on foreign-language vocabulary, in exactly the same way, to *names.*

Mr. Pukczyva's name is pronounced puck-shiv-a. Need I say more? Visualize a hockey puck shivering (it's on ice) and you've made that conglomeration of sound *meaningful* because it is *visual. Puck shiver* = Pukczyva.

You're introduced to Ms. Smolenski, ordinarily a zip name. But, see a *small lens* (camera) *ski*ing and the name no longer "zips."

Petrocelli (pet row jelly) (the *c* is a *ch* sound)

Bentavagnia (bent [weather] vane)

Van Nuys (van noise)

Carrasquillo (car *S* ski *O* [or oh], or car ass ski *O*)

Morales (more or less, or more Alice)

Jeffries (chef freeze/frees)

Cherofsky (sheriff ski, or chair off ski)

Ponchatrain (punch a train)

Cusack (cue sack)

McKenzie (me can see; Mack *N Z*)

Do you see? This is the first of three steps you will take toward a *phenomenal* memory for names *and* faces. Right now, I'm dealing with only names. When you're introduced to someone new, make his or her name *meaningful*, "seeable" in your mind, by coming up with a Substitute Word or Thought for it. Eventually, you'll be able to do this with any name, no matter its length or "difficulty." Break the long name into syllables if necessary, and the "meaning" will come to light. I met a Mr. Dimitriades. As I shook hands with him I thought of *the meat tree ate E's.* I know I'm being repetitive, but I had to (a) *hear* that name properly before I could come up with that Substitute Thought or picture; and (b) really think of, *concentrate on*, that name in order to apply the idea. And I did it all "without pain."

Many names already have meaning, names such as Brown, Taylor, Hart, Barnes, Hightower, Green, River(s), Freed, Lowe, Marsh, Piper, Plummer, Bloom, Sachs, Field(s), Gates, Bell, Glazer, Banks, Coffey, Holmes, Butler, Forrest, Knott, Baker, Cunningham, Gorman, Dewey, Katz, Pierce, Brooks, and Klinger, to name just a few.

The older you are, the more knowledge you've accrued. You may know that **Berg** means *mountain* in German, so you can visualize a mountain to represent that fairly common prefix or suffix. Or, you can choose to "see" an iceberg for that one. **Schoen** means *beautiful* and **Schneider** means *tailor* in German; **Noyer** means *walnut tree* in French, and so on. If you are familiar with these foreign words, they offer more options for attaching meaning to a name.

There's yet another category of names, those that have no specific meaning for you but conjure up an image. If you know baseball, **DiMaggio** would certainly make you visualize a baseball player, as would **Ruth**. **Caruso** might make you think of an opera singer. **Hudson** or **Jordan** might make you think of a river, **Campbell** might make you "see" a can of soup (or a "camp bell" might work better for you), **Graham** (gray ham) might bring the picture of a cracker to mind. Personal experience also works. When I hear the name **Browning**, I visualize a BAR, a Browning Automatic Rifle, with which I was quite familiar during World War II. A childhood friend named Elliott was a tennis nut. Whenever I hear the name **Elliott**, I think of tennis; Elliott reminds me of tennis, tennis reminds me of Elliott.

Now, to repeat that important point, the nitty-gritty of this whole chapter: What do you accomplish by applying the Substitute Word system to names?

You are forcing yourself to hear the name!

How could you possibly come up with *puck shiver* if you didn't hear, *make sure* you heard, *Pukczyva* in the first place? There's no way you can visualize yourself carrying a ton (carry ton) if you don't *hear* the name **Carrington** in the first place. So, you see, this whole strategy simply forces the application of **Rule 1: Be sure to hear the name.**

Apply the idea for a while and you'll start to form *standards*. For example, I *always* visualize a black*smith*'s hammer, or just a blacksmith for **Smith** (or **Schmidt**), a *garden* for **Gordon**, an ice-cream *cone* for **Cohen**. The same is true for common prefixes and suffixes. For **Mc** or **Mac** I see a Mack truck; for **ly** or **ley**, a meadow (lea); for **son**, son or sun; for **Berg, ice berg; ler**, law (perhaps a judge's gavel); for **witz** or **itz**, wits or itch; for **stein**, beer stein; for **ton**, the item weighs a ton; for **baum**, bum or bomb; for **ger**, grr (growling); and so on.

Remember that it's better for you to come up with your own Substitute Words or Thoughts, your own ridiculous pictures. My helping you in those areas isn't really helping you. When *I* suggest the word, thought, or phrase, *you* don't have to think, to concentrate on the name. Please keep that in mind. It's a difficult line for me to draw. I do want you to do that bit of thinking/concentrating because that's what locks in the name for you. On the other hand, I like to make some suggestions so that you realize how easy and obvious it all is. That's why I've given you quite a few examples. Here are a few more.

You might want to use these as a kind of drill—cover my suggestions with your hand or a piece of paper and see if you can come up with your own ideas. Then compare them to mine.

Kolamecko	collar make O	**Krakauer**	crack hour (clock)
Aldrich	old (and) rich	**Tropeano**	throw piano
Marquardt	Ma quart; mark what?	**Antesiewicz**	anti savage
Baldwin	bald one; bald win	**Halperin**	help her in
Baxter	back stir; back stair	**Abramson**	ram son
Anderson	hand and son; and her son	**Flanagan**	fan again
Evans	heavens; vans	**Michaels**	mike calls; Mike kills
Weber	web air; web bar	**Kessler**	cast law; kiss law
Talmadge	tall midget; tall Madge	**MacLeod**	my cloud; Mack loud
Shapiro	shape pear (O); chopper row	**Leonard**	lean hard
		Kennedy	can a day; can of Ds
Thompson	thump son; time son	**Patterson**	pat a son; batter son
Slocum	slow comb	**Reynolds**	rain holds; wren old
Webster	web stir; dictionary	**Rigney**	rig knee
Williams	will yams	**Nixon**	nicks on
		Rafferty	rap for tea

Try some on your own:

Padgett, Nussbaum, Abbott, Alexander, Cooper, Wellington, Simon, Bennett, Carson, Fleming, Crandall, Richards, Birnbaum, Allen, Malone, Lafferty, Mitchell, Monroe, Brewster, Frazer, Garrison.

It's a Given (Name)

Are you wondering, "What about first names?" I often get that question after I've taught how to handle surnames. My answer usually is, "What about them?" You can handle them exactly the same way. Come up with a Substitute Word or Thought for the first name exactly as you'd do for a surname.

And you'll be forming "standards" for first names, too, as you continue to apply the technique. For **Bill**, I always see a dollar bill— what else? For **Mary**, a wedding (*marry*); **George**, jaws or gorge; **Harry**, hairy or hurry; **Sylvia**, silver; **William**, will yam; **Bernard**, burn hard; **Tricia**, tree share; **James**, aims; **Tom** or **Thomas**, tom-tom drums or a tom cat; **Charles**, quarrels; **Susan**, sues Ann or sues ant; **Phillip**, full lip; **Tony**, toe knee; **Robert**, robber; **Howard**, coward; **Jim**, gym; **Jack**, carjack; **Anita**, an eater or anteater; **Mike**, mike (microphone); **Bernice**, burn knees; **Allen**, alley or a lens; and so forth.

Now think of a Substitute Word or Thought for the following on your own:

Bob, Caesar, Bruce, Byron, Clark, Wendy, Trudy, Sally, Phyllis, Ernie, Dennis, Douglas, Nancy, Molly, Ashley, Thelma, Ben, Harold, Gary, Richard, Victoria, Anthony, Adolph, Boris, Carl, Mel, Erwin, Mitchell, Fred, Daryl, Donald, Edward, Mildred, Millicent, Lillian, Gladys, Marcy, Alex, Andy, Eugene, Horace, Wallace, Vincent, Walter, Roxanne, John, Isabel.

Another question I get is: "Gee, if I think of a blacksmith's hammer for Smith every time I meet a Mr. or Mrs. Smith, won't that get confusing?" Absolutely not. Please remember that my techniques, tricks, methods, strategies (call them what you like) are *a means to an end*. When you meet a Mr. Smith and connect his face with a blacksmith's hammer, as you'll learn to do soon, you are locking in that name. And you're doing that with each Mr. Smith you meet. You are forcing yourself to hear the name, pay attention to the name, no matter how many times you use the same Substitute Thought. And the third or fourth time you see the same Mr. Smith, you'll *know his name*, his face will *tell* you his name. Your original mental "connection" will fade in direct ratio to how strongly that person's name becomes knowledge; you've reached the "end," the means are no longer needed!

Names and <u>more</u>

If you want to remember both the surname and the given name, include a Substitute Word or Thought for each in your mental image. If you like, you can also include something that will remind you that the person is, say, a doctor. You can include *whatever you like*.

Here's an example: You meet a Dr. Harry Gordon and you'd like to remember his full name and the fact that he's a doctor. Well, I would visualize a garden (Gordon) and there's *hair* covering much of the foliage and flowers—it's hairy (Harry), and there are some gigantic *stethoscopes* (or *one* giant stethoscope) growing in the garden. I always use a stethoscope to represent "doctor." Form this association when you meet and talk to Dr. Harry Gordon, and you've locked in not only his name but *more*. Effortlessly!

I've been the keynote speaker at a number of military functions. At some of them, everyone was in civilian clothes; at others, they were in uniform. When they were in civilian clothes, of course, I had no clue as to their rank, and when they were in uniform I *couldn't see* the bars or stars that'd tell me the rank anyway. But I wanted to remember not just people's names but their rank as well—so, for example, I used *loot* in my mental picture to tell me that the person was a lieutenant, a *cap* for captain, and a *gem* for general. Problem solved. Bear in mind that, at a speaking engagement, I meet and remember a few hundred people at one time. I have to be careful— you can't call a captain "Lieutenant" and you'd better not call a general anything but "General."

It is unlikely that you will ever have to remember hundreds of people at once, so it should be very easy for you to apply the technique successfully at any gathering.

Now It's Your Turn

When you agree that coming up with a Substitute Word or Thought for any name is easy (it's also *fun*) and when you understand the importance of doing so when meeting new people (you'll learn other uses, perhaps more important uses, for the idea as we go on), it's time to think about the second element: *faces*. We'll concentrate on those in the next chapter.

SPECIAL MIND-POWER EXERCISE #10

Grab four wooden matches (or toothpicks) and form the outline of a martini glass, as shown here. The *O* is the olive (or Gibson onion). Use a match head for that.

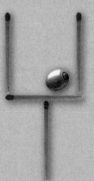

Here's the exercise: Move only *two* matches to bring the olive *outside* the glass.

You may *not* touch the olive, and the glass must end up shaped exactly as it was—it does not change shape at all. No, you do *not* break any matches.

It takes a bit of thinking—but that's the point, isn't it? Don't read the hint below until you've worked on this one a bit.

(Hint: The glass stays the same shape but it doesn't necessarily face the same direction.)

CHAPTER 11

Let's Face It

> "It is the common wonder of all men, how among so many millions of faces there should be none alike." —Sir Thomas Browne

"Oh, I recognize your face, but I don't remember your name."

During my long career I've heard this remark literally thousands of times. I've never heard it the other way around—I've never heard anyone say to someone they've met before, "I remember your name but I don't recognize your face"!

This makes perfect sense, because most of us are video minded as opposed to audio minded. That is, we remember what we see much better than what we hear. That's why my systems and techniques deal so much with that one concept, that one goal: to make anything we want to remember, whether heard or read, *meaningful*—so that we can visualize it in our minds, see it in our mind's eye, and consequently remember it.

So, when it comes to names and faces, why not take advantage of the fact that it is the face we usually recognize? My method for remembering names and faces does exactly that, as well as it will ever get done, for everyone, but particularly for mature people. A lady in her eighties once told me that she had many grandchildren and was starting to have trouble remembering all of their names. She learned and started to apply the system I'm teaching here and—problem solved. Now she uses the technique on everyone, from waiters, waitresses, plumbers, and carpenters to the butcher, the baker, and the candlestick maker. She's become a local celebrity: everyone knows her name because she knows everyone else's!

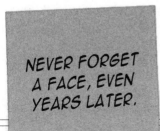

NEVER FORGET A FACE, EVEN YEARS LATER.

All right then, let's move on. You've already applied the first step, which you learned in the preceding chapters—that is, you heard the name and decided on a Substitute Word or Thought in order to make that name meaningful. Now, look at the person's face and select what you think is the *outstanding feature* on that face.

It can be anything: high forehead, low forehead, creases in the forehead, hairline, bald head, thin eyebrows, thick eyebrows, arched eyebrows, close-set eyes, wide-set eyes, big or small ears, outstanding ears, large earlobes, big nose, full cheeks, sunken cheeks, wide mouth, mustache, beard, thin lips, thick or full lips, large or small chin, cleft in chin, wrinkles, warts, pimples, dimples— anything. What you select may not be what someone else would select as the outstanding feature, but that doesn't matter. It's what's outstanding to *you* that matters.

When I'm teaching this at a corporate seminar I sometimes ask the people to look at my face and shout out the outstanding feature. I hear as many as six or seven different ones, and that's okay; that's as it should be. (It's usually the lines on my forehead. We used to call them "worry" lines; now they're "character" lines!)

What's important is that, to decide on the outstanding feature, you have to do what 99 percent of us don't habitually do: that is, look— *really look*— at that face! Listen, if I could invent a machine that you could place on your head, which would *automatically force you* to listen and look, I'd sell millions of them. Unfortunately, there is no such machine, so my system for remembering names and faces has to take its place. This is what I mean when I say that even if my systems didn't work, they'd still work. Do you see? There's no way to apply my system without *really listening and looking*. To come up with the Substitute Word or Thought, you must really *listen* so that you hear the name, and to select an outstanding facial feature, you must really *look* at that face. So, even if my systems didn't work, you'd have bettered your memory for names and faces by a high percentage. But my systems have been proven to work—and to give you a memory for names and faces beyond your wildest dreams!

Now you've just learned the second of the three steps, so let's review: **Step 1: Form a Substitute Word or Thought for the name. Step 2:**

Select an outstanding feature of the face. Fine, you're doing well. Let's move on to the third step, the step that will make the face (which you usually recognize anyway) *tell* you the name that goes with it!

Step 3 is simply to *connect* Steps 1 and 2. That's it. Connect your Substitute Word or Thought for the name to the outstanding feature of the face. It's obvious, right? You want one to remind you of the other. There are those two entities again.

I've used Mr. Bentavagnia as an example before. He seems to lock in the idea for people just learning it, so I'll use him again now. You've just been introduced to Mr. Bentavagnia. You listen to the name and apply Step 1, thinking of a *bent* (weather) *vane*. Then you move on to Step 2 and *look* at Mr. Bentavagnia's face.You see a large, bulbous nose, which you immediately select as the outstanding facial feature. Finally, you connect the two things via the use of a silly, ridiculous mental picture, as you've already learned to do. As you shake hands with Mr. Bentavagnia, and as you're looking at his face, "see" a *bent vane* on his face *instead of a nose*! That's it and that's all. There are different ways to "look" at it, of course. For example, you could have "seen" many bent vanes coming out of the nostrils of that "outstanding" nose. Either association is good, as long as you've connected the two entities, the name and the face.

You can practice this by assigning made-up names to pictures of faces in newspapers and magazines. Apply the system you've just learned to a few pictures, then go back and see if you know/ remember those names. I don't really like the "practice" concept, since your best practice is to just do it—but this really isn't practice, it's a *mind exercise*. From now on, you can use the system for real, with the new people you meet. You'll start to see results right away. You have absolutely nothing to lose, of course, since you've been forgetting names—or should I say *not remembering* names—all your life. The worst that can happen is that my system won't work for you. You'll just be in the same place you've always been in. So go ahead, apply the system. You'll amaze yourself.

Let's try something. You've just met Big Nose = Bentavagnia. Really see the "Bentavagnia" picture in your mind. Now meet Ms. Ponchatrane. You listen to the name and think *punch a train*. You look at her face and decide that her large ears are the outstanding facial feature. You "see" trains coming out of those ears and you punch one of them. Please, *see* that silly picture because I want you to prove something to yourself in a moment or two. Large Ears = Ponchatrane.

Mr. Pukczyva has an obvious cleft in his chin. As you shake hands with him, and say, "How d'ya do," you see many hockey pucks flying out of that cleft and they're icy and shivering; *puck shiver*. You can see the pucks tearing the cleft apart, if you want to. I told you, violence is the most ridiculous for me, and the "ridiculouser" the better. That's Cleft Chin = Pukczyva. Really *see* the picture.

Mr. Robrum has very bushy eyebrows. See a bottle of rum over each eye instead of eyebrows, and you "rob" them. Bushy Eyebrows = Robrum. *See* that silly picture.

Feel free to review the names and faces in your mind, as you would do if you were meeting a whole group of real people. There's nothing wrong with that. Look at the faces again and see if the names come to mind. Go over the four "people" you just met. Then we'll meet a few more.

Mr. Cohen has deep creases from his nostrils to the corners of his mouth. You've selected those creases as the outstanding facial feature. Really *see* dripping ice-cream cones coming out of those creases. Facial creases = Cohen.

The first thing you notice on Mr. Fleming's face is his large mustache. See it burning, *flaming*. Mustache = Fleming. Really *see* that mental image.

Ms. Cantrowitz has a large wart at the corner of her mouth. See brains (wits) coming out of that wart; you try to throw away those wits, but you can't. Can't throw wits = Cantrowitz. You must *see* that silly picture.

You're introduced to Mr. Smith. You think of a blacksmith's hammer and you decide to connect that to his obvious (to you) thick lips. I would see the blacksmith's hammer hammering those lips, which is what's making them so thick. Thick lips = Smith. Be particularly sure to *see* this silly mental image, because the tendency when meeting a Jones or a Smith is to think, "Oh, there's no way I'll forget an easy name like that; no need to bother with a mental picture." And then, of course, that *is* the one you don't remember. And that's more embarrassing than if you didn't remember a name like Katzenberger-Boyd! (*Cats* eating a *burger* and giving some to a *bird*.) So always be sure to "systemize" even a seemingly "easy" name.

One more: The outstanding feature on Mr. Kirschenberg's face is his very high forehead. "See" an iceberg coming out of that forehead, or an iceberg *instead of* a forehead, and you're *cursin'* it. Cursin' berg = Kirschenberg. This is the last "test" name; be sure to see your ridiculous association.

Test Time

You've carefully pictured the mental images I suggested, so if I were to mention one of the names we've learned, you'd probably find it easy to come up with the accompanying facial feature. For example, if I said "Fleming," you'd think, "A large mustache is flaming." But in real life, it has to work the other way around. The point is not that the name should remind you of the face but that the face must remind you of the name. And since first impressions are lasting impressions, the outstanding feature you selected will be outstanding to you when you see that face again.

As a good test, I've listed the outstanding facial features below, just as if I were showing you an actual picture of the face or as if you were seeing that face at a social or business gathering. Put the correct name into each blank.

Bushy eyebrows = _____ Thick lips = _____

Large ears = _____ High forehead = _____

Mustache = _____ Big bulbous nose = _____

Large wart = _____ Cleft chin = _____

Deep creases nose to mouth corners = _____

How'd you do? Forgive the redundancy, but if you goofed on one or two, go back, strengthen your mental picture, your association of the two entities, and try again.

A Boost to What You Already Have

I'm often asked by someone who has yet to apply this system in real life, "But what if I see Mr. Robrum again and, yes, the bushy eyebrows reminds me of 'robbing rum,' but I call him Mr. *Rumrob* instead of Mr. Robrum?"

The answer is that this simply won't happen because *true memory* tells you the correct name. Remember that my systems are simply *aids* to your true and fabulous God-given memory. There's no way you'd call Mr. Kirschenberg Mr. Bergenkirsch! It just wouldn't happen. And you know, I think Mr. Robrum would be happier if you called him Rumrob than if you called him "Hey" or "Buddy" or "Mac" or "Fella"! I usually end my response to this question by saying, "Please don't create problems where none exist."

In Conclusion

Herald Price Fahringer is a good-looking, white-haired gentleman and a renowned criminal lawyer. He uses my memory systems all the time, socially and in his work. He's written articles in law journals about me and my techniques. Here's a quote from Mr. Fahringer: "In the practice of law I use Harry Lorayne's system every day. I use it to remember names of jurors, I use it to remember names of important cases, I use it to remember items on a check list—dates, facts, places, times. Without it I would be lost."

Applying my technique *will definitely* better your memory for names and faces. I know, because I practice what I preach! Think about it: have you ever really seen Evelyn Wood read quickly? Have you ever seen Dale Carnegie make friends and influence people? Of course not. But I've demonstrated the ability to remember names and faces using my own systems over the years on major television shows all over the world (including twenty times on *The Tonight Show* with Johnny Carson). And as you have no doubt figured out, I am considerably over 50 myself. Over the years, students of mine have demonstrated the skills I've taught them publicly, too.

Here's a guarantee: The first time you try my system for remembering names and faces when in a small group of people, you'll remember 50 percent more names than you ever did before. The second time you try it you'll remember 75 percent more, and the third time—100 percent more!

I know exactly what I'm doing, of course. The only way you can prove me wrong is by *trying it* at least three times. So, do it—you have nothing to lose!

SPECIAL MIND-POWER EXERCISE #11

This is an oldie but a goody, and it will give your mind a bit of a workout. Some thinking is involved here, so be patient.

The challenge is to connect all the dots in the square layout below using only *four straight lines*, and without lifting your pen or pencil from the paper.

Remember, you cannot lift your pencil off the paper. You may *not* touch any dot more than once (and there's no folding involved).

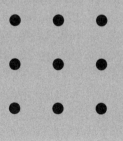

CHAPTER 12

I <u>See</u> Numbers!

POETTARRARORINCOAROAC

According to the *Guinness Book of World Records*, the above is the word for "three" among the primitive people of the Yancos, an Amazon tribe. It's as high as they count. Imagine if they had to remember the numbers up to ten!

We have to remember numbers into the millions and billions.

Do something for me, would you? Look at this number and this sentence for only a moment or two; say each to yourself.

0147271326390092112

A STARK NAKED MAN JUMPS UP AND DOWN.

Good. I'll get back to them shortly.

Everyone agrees that the two most difficult-to-remember areas are names and faces, and numbers. When I'm called on to do seminars for corporations I always ask, What are the two kinds of things you would like your people to remember better? No matter what the business is, the answer is *always* names and numbers, numbers and names.

REMEMBERING NUMBERS IN A BRAND-NEW WAY.

The reason, of course, is that names and numbers are *abstract* concepts. You now know how to make names tangible, meaningful. Numbers are at the head of the class here because they are completely abstract, they are only designs on paper, and what do they actually mean in your mind? What does 7 mean to you except that it's one less than 8 and one higher than 6?

I can't help but think that the system I'm about to teach you for remembering numbers (to a degree you never dreamed possible) will be the most important new thing you'll learn here. The idea is applicable to so many other problems, so many other areas, it can literally change your life, as many have so advised me. But, let's take it one step at a time.

The Phonetic Alphabet

The first step in remembering numbers is to learn a new "alphabet," the *Phonetic Alphabet*. No need to panic; it consists of only ten units and I'll give you a strong memory aid for each one. You had to learn and remember twenty-six shapes and sounds (the abc's) when you were a young child, and with no memory aids. With the memory aids I'll give you, this will be child's play for you. As a matter of fact, I teach it to children and they know it in minutes.

There are, of course, only ten digits in our number system: 1, 2, 3, 4, 5, 6, 7, 8, 9, and 0. What you need to learn is ten simple sounds, each one of which will represent one of our numerical digits. Fortunately, there are also only ten *basic* consonant sounds in our language. (Technically there are more, but there's no need for us to get technical; we need only the ten basic consonant sounds, as you'll see.)

You're going to connect a digit to a sound, and vice versa, and those pairs will always remain the same—so once learned, forever beneficial, forever used.

It's the sound that's important, not the letter or letters used to form that sound, because different letters make the same sound.

There's an old gag that says GHOTI is another way to spell FISH. The GH as in "enou*gh*," the O as in "w*o*men" and the TI as in "mo*ti*on." It's a joke but it's true. The point is that the *gh* and *f* make the same consonant sound in these examples, as do *ti* and *sh*. And so do *t* and *d*; *p* and *b*; *ph, v,* and *f; j, ch, sh,* and soft *g* (as in *g*ent); *s* and soft *c* (as in *c*ent); *k*, hard *c* (as in *c*oat), and hard *g* (as in *g*oat). If your vocal apparatus, your lips, tongue, and teeth, are all in the same position to sound out two or three different letters or letter combinations (like *j* and *sh*) they are the *same consonant sound.* Okay, here are the ten pairs and your memory aid for each one. Pay attention to each memory aid; think of it, see it, in your mind.

1 = t (and by extension d)
The typewritten *t* has *one* downstroke; or, a horizontal 1 on top of a vertical 1 forms a *t*.

2 = n
The typewritten lower-case n has *two* downstrokes.

3 = m
The typewritten lower-case m has *three* downstrokes. Or, think of the 3M Corporation; or, if you stand a lower-case m on its side it becomes a 3.

4 = r
Think of, and stress, the final sound of fou*r*. Or, look at a capital letter *R*: using a bit of imagination, can you see a golfer about to drive? And, what does he shout as he is about to take his swing? "Fore!"

5 = l
The Roman numeral L is *50*. Or, hold up your open left hand, fingers together, thumb extended to the right, as if signaling "stop," and you're forming a capital letter *L* with your *five* fingers.

6 = j (and also sh, ch, soft g)
The digit 6 and the capital letter *J* are almost mirror images. (**LJ**)

7 = k (as well as hard c, hard g)
You can form a capital letter *K* with two 7s, one right side up, the other upside down. (**K**)

8 = f (and v, ph)
An 8 and a small handwritten script *f* each have one loop above the other. Put a tail between the two loops of the 8 and it looks like the

handwritten small *f*.

9 = p (also b)
The 9 and *P* are just about mirror images. (**9P**)

0 = s (as well as soft c, z)
Think of the first sound in the word *z*ero or the first sound in the word *c*ipher.

That's the Phonetic Alphabet:

1 = t or d	6 = j, sh, ch, soft g
2 = n	7 = k, hard g, hard c
3 = m	8 = f, v, ph
4 = r	9 = p, b
5 = l	0 = s, soft c, z

  That's all there is to it. If you've paid even a small bit of attention to the memory aids I've suggested, you now *know* the Phonetic Alphabet. If you haven't paid attention to the memory aids, go back and do so now. Then, fill in the following blanks:

1 ___ 2 ___ 3 ___ 4 ___ 5 ___ 6 ___ 7 ___ 8 ___ 9 ___ 0 ___

2 ___ 4 ___ 6 ___ 8 ___ 0 ___ 9 ___ 7 ___ 5 ___ 3 ___ 1 ___

n ___ j ___ r ___ p ___ l ___ t ___ k ___

m ___ s ___ f ___ sh ___ g as in *go* ___ ph ___

0 ___ 9 ___ 8 ___ 7 ___ 6 ___ 5 ___ 4 ___ 3 ___ 2 ___ 1 ___

If you filled in all the blanks, you know the sounds and the digits they represent in and out of order, backward, forward, inside out and every which way. Believe me, after just a bit of use, they will become second nature, ingrained, as is the 26-letter alphabet.

(Actually, even more so. If I asked you to tell me the, say, 13th letter of our regular alphabet, you'd have to count on your fingers. In the Phonetic Alphabet, no finger counting is necessary, as there are only ten sounds.)

And those ten "connections" are all you need—except for a few rules. And a few answers to your inevitable questions. (I'm anticipating your questions, because they won't really come up until you actually start to apply the concept.) The vowels *a, e, i, o, u,* by themselves, have no value at all, nor do the letters *w, h,* and *y* (the "old vowels"). The *h,* of course, changes the sound of other letters, as when it follows immediately after a *g* or a *c.* The vowels are the "glue" that connects the consonants, as you'll see.

Silent letters have no value because they make no sound! The word "knee," for example, makes only the one *n* sound, because the *k* is not sounded. Of course, if someone speaks with an accent, and does pronounce or sound that *k,* then it *would* have value, the value of 7. "Bomb" makes only two consonant sounds, *b* then *m*; the final *b* is silent.

For our purposes, the *th* sound is the same as *t*; it represents the digit 1. *Q* usually makes the *k* sound so it represents the digit 7. *X* will rarely come up, but for the sake of completeness, it represents the sound it makes in the particular word. In "anxious," it makes a *k/sh* sound, which is 7, 6. In "xylophone" it's either *g/z* (7, 0) or just 0, depending on how *you* pronounce it.

Double letters make one sound. The *tt* in "butter" makes one *t* sound (you don't say "butiter") so it represents 1, not 11. Butter = 914. The *nn* in "banner" makes one *n* sound. Banner = 924; pillow = 95; callous = 750.

Okay. Time for a bit of practice:

borrow _____   manly _____   suffer _____   car _____   automobile _____

chandelier _____   sorrow _____   attention _____   chiropractor _____

turpentine _____   sure _____   chair _____   tangerine _____

Here are the number groups you should have put into the blanks: borrow = 94, manly = 325, suffer = 084, car = 74, automobile = 1395, chandelier = 62154, sorrow = 04, attention = 1262, chiropractor = 7494714, turpentine = 149212, sure = 64, chair = 64, tangerine = 12642.

Did you convert "chandelier" correctly? The word "attention" could have been a double trap for you. Check them all out and if you were wrong on any, make sure you understand *why* you were wrong.

What's the Idea?

Now, you're wondering, "Okay, so I know the Phonetic Alphabet, I know the digits that the consonant sounds represent. What good does it do me? How do I apply this knowledge? Well, let's see if this answers that question for you, and impresses you in the process. Do you remember that I asked you to look at a long number and a sentence at the top of this chapter? Please don't look back at them now. Do you remember the long number? When I reach this point at personal seminars and ask this question I get laughs and remarks like, "Are you kidding?"

My next question is, "Do you remember the sentence?" Most do. Well...if you know that sentence you also know the long number! That is, you know it because of what you just learned: the Phonetic Alphabet. Look:

A <u>stark naked man jumps up and down.</u>

0147 271 32 6390 9 21 12
(014727132639092112)

I see eyes widen when I do this on the blackboard at a corporate seminar. I hope I've gotten a similar reaction from you.

Understand, please, that trying to find either silly or familiar sentences (Mary had a little lamb = 34151553; a pretty girl is like a melody = 941745057351) is silly and time wasting. I used the sentence only as a *teaching device*. It works *the other way around*.

I need to stress what should be obvious to you now. The Phonetic Alphabet enables you to *make numbers meaningful*, visual in your mind! How in the world would you ordinarily visualize, say, 147? Now, you can "see" a *truck*, which can represent *only* 147. Part of the beauty of the concept is that there are *no decisions to make*. It's a definite. Truck, trick, track, drake, drag, dark, derrick, turkey— each of these represent 147; there's no way any of them could represent anything *but* 147 in our Phonetic Alphabet.

Assume you want to remember 147 275 952 127. Apply what you've just learned—the Phonetic Alphabet—*and* the idea you learned some chapters ago, the Link system of memory. Look at the number, which I've broken into groups of three only for teaching purposes. We've already talked about the first part, 147. Simply think the sounds to yourself: *trk...truck*. "See" a truck.

Look at the next three digits and "sound them out": 275 is *nkl... nickel* comes to mind. *Knuckle, uncle, ankle* would also fit, but assume that *nickel* comes to mind first. Start a Link by connecting *truck* to *nickel*. You might see millions of nickels pouring out of a truck, or a gigantic nickel *is* a truck, or a gigantic nickel is driving a truck, etc. *See* the picture you select.

Moving on to 952: *pln* or *bln*. *Balloon* can represent only 952. So make *nickel* remind you of *balloon*. You can see yourself blowing up a nickel instead of a balloon, or a child is holding a large nickel on a string instead of a balloon, etc. I could go on and on, but you need only one ridiculous picture. Choose one and *see* it in your mind: nickel to balloon.

Now, 127: *tnk, tank*. (*Dunk, think, dank, tang, tunic* would also fit.) Make *balloon* remind you of *tank*. Millions of balloons are flying out of a tank, you're blowing up a tank instead of a balloon, hundreds of balloons are lifting a tank into the air, whatever. *See* the picture you select.

By Linking just four items, you've remembered a 12-digit number! Think of *truck*. What does *truck* remind you of? *Nickel*, of course. *Nickel*, in turn, makes you think of *balloon*. And *balloon* reminds you of *tank*. Truck-nickel-balloon-tank. Just transpose the consonants to digits:

Truck nickel balloon tank = 147 275 952 127

You know that you can "do" a Link backward, not that you'd ever have to or want to, except to show off. But if you can do a Link backward, you can also do a long-digit number backward. Try it so that you can see how well it "works." Think of the last item of your Link, *tank*. Thinking backward, the digits are 721. Tank makes you think of *balloon;* think the digits backward, 259. Balloon reminds you of *nickel*, that's 572 backward, and, finally, nickel reminds you of *truck,* which is 741 backward. The entire number—backward—is 721259572741. Wow!

A simple four-word Link and you've memorized a twelve-digit number. I'm stressing this because, according to some Intelligence Quotient tests, an adult of average intelligence can remember a six-digit number forward and backward after hearing or seeing it once. An adult with *superior* intelligence can do the same with an eight-digit number. You've just done it with a *twelve*-digit number! There's no "category" for you! And there's no limit to your mind's ability to retain information.

Realistically, if this was a number that was important to you, one that you *used*, then after three or four uses, it'd become knowledge. But it's okay to think of your Link to remind you of it, and it does that beautifully, plus affording some mental exercise.

Personally, I would have "locked in" that number with a quick *three*-word Link: truck, nickel *planting* = 147 275 952127. Whenever I see 27 in a long number I try to tack *ing* onto the preceding word. That *ing* always represents 27 to me. When I see a zero, I pluralize the preceding word with an *s*. So, if the example number had been 1470275952127, I would have Linked *trucks-nickel-planting*.

Are you with me? Would you like to remember a number as long as this one?

2859495240169520715191196

If you worked with me back in chapter 5 and did the sample Link starting with *envelope* and ending with *shoe*, you've already memorized it! A 25-digit number!

Look at this ordinarily formidable number: 9483158295147412. Let's break it down, again for teaching purposes, into groups of four: 9483 1582 9514 7412. Work with me. Think *prfm*, perfume; *tlfn*, telephone; *bltr*, blotter; *krtn*, carton. Link *perfume* to *telephone* to *blotter* to *carton*, and you've memorized a sixteen-digit number pretty quickly. Obviously, the better you know your sounds, the faster and more easily you'll remember numbers.

Keep in mind that in "real life" I never break numbers into even groups this way. You could have looked at 9483158295147412 and thought: bear-fumed-livin' (or lovin') up-letter-car-tin. Or, brave-medal-fan-belt-rock-rotten. When I want to "do" a number quickly, as a show-off thing or a demonstration, I use the first things that come to mind. When it's a number I need in my real life, I take a bit more time to think of longer, perhaps, better words, objects, pictures.

Try some on your own. No need to do them all at the same time. Rest in between, as you would when doing any exercise.

994 614 757 954 (You can start your Link with paper or piper.)

4210 5214 6127 9071 (Rents can start your Link.)

522 641 639 527 (Linen is a good start.)

9427 9205 5210 7412
(Bring, praying, boring, pouring, and brink are all good starts.)

After you've "done" these, and what a great mental exercise they are, rewrite the numbers without spaces, without breaking them into a pattern, and see what other words you can come up with to fit them. That's another great mental exercise. Who ever said we get dull as we age?

We have come a long way in this chapter! If you've made it your business to really know the sounds of the Phonetic Alphabet, we can go on to some more practical uses for the technique. We are not finished with numbers by a long shot.

Now I'm going to talk to you about *Pegs*.

SPECIAL MIND-POWER EXERCISE #12

Let's make a couple of assumptions. You have a regular scale (not a "balance" scale) that registers weight in both ounces and grams.

You also have five bags, each containing fifteen coins; each coin weighs one ounce, so the bag of fifteen coins weighs fifteen ounces. Except—all of the coins in one of the bags are counterfeit; each of the coins in that bag weighs one gram less than a full ounce. (The counterfeit coins look exactly like the legitimate coins, of course.)

Here's your problem, and your mind exercise. You're allowed only *one* weighing, during which you can weigh whatever you like. You can weigh one bag, two, three, four, or all five at one time.

So, do one weighing, however you like—and determine which bag holds the fifteen counterfeit coins.

Yes, it can be done logically.

CHAPTER 13

Peg(s) O' My Heart

"We are born unarmed. Our mind is our only weapon." —Ayn Rand

If you try to hang your coat on a flat wall, it will fall to the ground. Put a short peg into that wall and you have something onto which to hang that coat. I'm not interested in your wall or coat, I'm interested in your mind and memory—so I'll give you "pegs" for your mind, pegs upon which you can "hang" thoughts and information. I call it the Peg System of Memory, and it's based on what you already know, the consonant sounds of the Phonetic Alphabet.

You know how to apply the Link System to remember items in sequence which, of course, is terrific. But what if, for whatever reason, you need to know the items in *and* out of order, by number? If you wanted to know what the, say, sixth item was, you'd have to go over your Link, counting on your fingers or counting mentally until you got to the item. What you're about to learn is a simple method that solves that problem. It enables you to remember any kind of information *by number.*

Let's start by learning Peg Words. They're easy to remember because of their familiar sounds. The simple concept is that the word must contain *only* the consonant sound(s) that represents that number in the Phonetic Alphabet you already know. So, the Peg Word for #1 can contain only the *t* sound.

HANDLING MORE CHALLENGING NUMBERS AS NEVER BEFORE.

The word I've selected for #1, and always use, is *tie*. Make sure that you understand why. And of course I always select words that can be easily visualized. For *tie*, obviously, you'd visualize a necktie. *Tie* will always represent, can *only* represent, the #1.

The Peg Word for #2 is **Noah**. Again, be sure you understand why Noah can only represent #2. (Remember the Phonetic Alphabet.) Visualize an old man with a beard on an ark, or just the ark.

#3 is **Ma**. Visualize your mother.

#4 is **rye**. Picture a bottle of rye whiskey or a loaf of rye bread.

#5 is **law**. The word "law," on its own, cannot easily be visualized, so "see" something that *represents* law to you, a policeman or a judge's gavel, for example.

#6 is **shoe**. Easy enough, picture a shoe. Do you see why **shoe** can represent *only* the single digit, 6? Of course, because it contains only the *sh* sound which, as you know, is 6 in the Phonetic Alphabet.

#7 is **cow**. See a cow—what else?

#8 is **ivy**; it contains only the one consonant sound *v* and that is 8. Picture ivy clinging to or climbing on a wall.

#9 is **bee**. See a bee, of course.

#10 has two digits, so the Peg Word for 10 must contain *two* consonant sounds: *t* for 1 and *s* for 0, in that order. The Peg Word is **toes**; do you understand why? Picture toes.

Those are the first ten Peg Words. They're easy to remember because knowing the sound(s) the word must contain practically tells you what it is. You'll be amazed at how quickly you'll know them and how soon you'll be able to actually count using the words instead of numbers! And, because you know the sounds out of order, you also know the Peg Words out of order. Right now, look at the first ten Peg Words in order once more.

1	tie	6	shoe
2	Noah	7	cow
3	Ma	8	ivy
4	rye	9	bee
5	law	10	toes

Now, fill in these blanks.

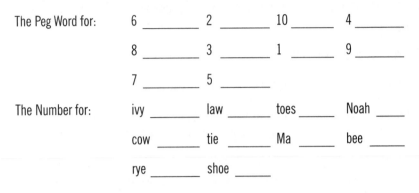

The Peg Word for: 6 _____   2 _____   10 _____   4 _____

8 _____   3 _____   1 _____   9 _____

7 _____   5 _____

The Number for: ivy _____   law _____   toes _____   Noah ____

cow _____   tie _____   Ma _____   bee _____

rye _____   shoe _____

Using Peg Words

You might want to let these first ten Peg Words sink in for a while before you go to the next step, which is a basic application of the words. When you feel you're ready, I'll show you how to use them. Ready? Okay. I'll give you ten items in a completely haphazard order, by number, with a quick suggestion for your association. Now you can visualize the numbers from 1 to 10 because you've given them meaning—that's the whole point.

Let's assume that for some reason you have to remember that #5 is *fork*. See either a gigantic fork in a cop's uniform, walking his beat (upholding the *law*), or a judge banging a gigantic fork instead of a gavel. Be sure to *see* the silly picture.

#8 is *pen*. Millions of pens are growing on a brick wall instead of *ivy* or you're writing on a wall of ivy with a gigantic pen. See ink dripping all over the ivy. Select one of these pictures or one you think of yourself, and *see* it in your mind's eye.

#1 is *pillow*. You might see yourself wearing a large pillow instead of a *tie*. Or a large pillow is wearing a tie, or your head is resting on many neckties instead of on a pillow. Be sure to *see* the ridiculous picture.

#6 is *computer*. You're wearing computers on your feet instead of *shoe*s; a large computer is wearing shoes and walking; a gigantic shoe is typing at the computer. Use one of these silly pictures and *see* it.

#9 is *scissors*. See many scissors buzzing around you and stinging you like *bee*s. Or, millions of bees are attacking you and you're cutting those bees in half with a gigantic pair of scissors. *See* it.

You might want to go back over these first five before continuing.

#3 is *flower*. You might see a gigantic flower holding a baby—it's a *Ma*. Or, your mother is a gigantic flower, or your mother is holding a gigantic flower between her teeth, or she is growing in a garden like a flower. There are so many ways to go; all you need to do is visualize one ridiculous picture.

#10 is *DVD*. There's a DVD between all your *toes*, or each toe is a DVD, or you're placing a gigantic toe into your DVD player. *See* that picture.

#4 is *car*. See a gigantic bottle of *rye* whiskey driving a car, or a car is drinking rye whiskey, or each wheel of a car is a bottle of rye whiskey. Or, use rye bread instead of the bottle of rye. Whichever you're using, *see* the picture.

#7 is *egg*. Imagine yourself milking a gigantic egg instead of a *cow*, or you're milking a cow and many eggs come out instead of milk, etc. *See* that picture.

#2 is *Benadryl*. I'm using this on purpose to show you that now you can remember an abstract thing because you know the Substitute Word technique. For this you might see an old man with a white beard (or whatever you're "seeing" to represent *Noah*) bending a drill—*bend a drill*, Benadryl. Or, bent drills are boarding the ark two by two. Be sure to see this last picture in your mind. If you think you need a quick review, do so. Then, fill in these blanks:

#1 (tie) is _____	#6 (shoe) is _____
#2 (Noah) _____	#7 (cow) is _____
#3 (Ma) is _____	#8 (ivy) is _____
#4 (rye) is _____	#9 (bee) is _____
#5 (law) is _____	#10 (toes) is _____

Impressed? It gets better. You "heard" ten items in a completely haphazard order and you just listed them in order, 1 to 10, and that's great—your mind is starting to work like a computer! And you know those ten items forward, backward, upside down, inside out, in any order. Try this:

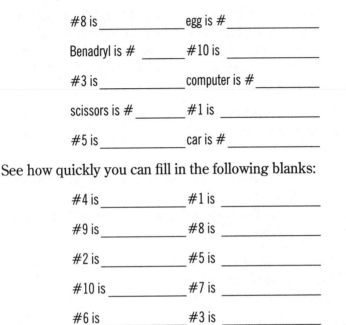

#8 is _____ egg is # _____

Benadryl is # _____ #10 is _____

#3 is _____ computer is # _____

scissors is # _____ #1 is _____

#5 is _____ car is # _____

See how quickly you can fill in the following blanks:

#4 is _____ #1 is _____

#9 is _____ #8 is _____

#2 is _____ #5 is _____

#10 is _____ #7 is _____

#6 is _____ #3 is _____

You've done something with your memory, your mind, that you never did or could do before—and that "youngsters," people much younger than you are, *can't do* (unless they know my memory-training systems).

Getting Practical

You can use this as a show-off thing in front of friends and family (and, more important, as a great mind exercise) but—even better—you can also use it for *practical* purposes: the items can be errands or appointments throughout your day. You can, of course, remember errands and appointments in order via the Link system, but now, if you prefer, you can memorize them by number. That's your call: #6 ("computer") might be your reminder to buy a new mouse for your home computer; #2 ("Benadryl") could be your reminder to pick up your prescription; #7 ("egg") might be your reminder to pick up a dozen eggs, and so forth. We'll be discussing *practical* applications much more as we continue on our road to a much, much better memory.

Right now, you can remember items by number because you know ten Peg Words. But what if you wanted or needed to remember *eleven* things, or twelve, or twenty, by number? Simply learn Peg Words from 11 to 20! Wouldn't it be great if all problems were this easy to solve? It's easy because of the Phonetic Alphabet. The sounds practically tell you the words. Here they are:

11	tide	16	dish
12	tin	17	dog
13	tomb	18	dove
14	tire	19	tub
15	tail	20	nose

You see why each word "fits" phonetically, right? For *tin*, see item #12 as made of tin (or, as I do, always visualize a tin can); see a tombstone for *tomb*; the others are pretty much self-explanatory. Go over them once or twice. When you're ready, here's my test and your mind exercise. Fill in the blanks with the proper Peg Word.

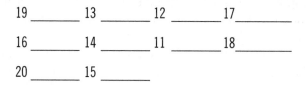

19 _____ 13 _____ 12 _____ 17 _____

16 _____ 14 _____ 11 _____ 18 _____

20 _____ 15 _____

Learn these first twenty Peg Words, make them second nature; of course, this will happen automatically as you *use* them. Now you can show off for friends and family. Write down numbers from 1 to 20 (or 1 to 15) on a piece of paper. Have your friends call out numbers and random items. Ask one of them to write in each item next to its corresponding number (because they won't remember them!), which also gives you the bit of time you may need to make your association. When all of the numbers have items written next to them, let your friends test you. You can call off the items in order, then out of order. Have someone call out any number and you say the item; have someone else call out an item and you say the number.

And, yes, you can use your Peg Words over and over, whether you're showing off for fun, as above, or using them for practical purposes or just mental exercise. It's like a child's magic slate toy: when the top plastic sheet is lifted, all the writing disappears and you're left with a blank slate, ready to use again.

You can, of course, learn up to 100 Peg Words, though you may never need them (and if you do need them, you can easily make them up as needed). Once you make up a word for a number, that's the word that will always come back to you. They come in handy in many different situations, the least of which is that you find you need to know (remember) that a certain thing is #73. In that case you would simply associate that "thing" to *comb*. If you do that, and if you know your sounds, there is no way you'll experience that darn "senior moment" that makes you say or think, "What the heck number was that 'thing'? It went right out of my mind." No more. When you think of that "thing" and it's "connected" to *comb*, you simply *know* that it's #73.

Peg Words also come in handy when memorizing a long-digit number and you're stuck at two digits, or when it's better to "do" two digits as, for example, in learning your social security number. The middle grouping is always two digits, e.g., _ _ _ 42 _ _ _ _ . You might want to use a word or phrase for the first three digits, then *rain* for the 42, then a word or phrase for the final four digits. Again, it's your choice. Here are the Peg Words I've used for decades.

1. tie	26. notch	51. lot	76. cage
2. Noah	27. neck	52. lion	77. coke
3. Ma	28. knife	53. lame (loom)	78. cave
4. rye	29. knob	54. lure	79. cap (cob)
5. law	30. mouse	55. lily	80. fuzz (face)
6. shoe	31. mat	56. leech (lash)	81. fit (fat)
7. cow	32. moon	57. lake (log)	82. phone (fan)
8. ivy	33. mummy	58. leaf (lava)	83. foam
9. bee	34. mower	59. lip (lap)	84. fur (fire)
10. toes	35. mule	60. cheese	85. file (foal)
11. tide (tot)	36. match	61. sheet	86. fish
12. tin	37. mug	62. chain	87. fog (fake)
13. tomb	38. movie	63. chum (jam)	88. fife
14. tire	39. mop	64. cherry	89. fob
15. tail (towel)	40. rose	65. jail (shell)	90. bus
16. dish	41. rod (root)	66. choo-choo	91. bat (boat)
17. dog (tack)	42. rain	67. chalk (jack)	92. bone (pan)
18. dove	43. ram	68. chef (chief)	93. bum (beam)
19. tub	44. rower (roar)	69. ship	94. bear (bar)
20. nose	45. roll (rail)	70. case	95. bell (ball)
21. net	46. roach (rash)	71. cot (coat)	96. beach
22. nun	47. rock	72. coin	97. book (bug)
23. name (gnome)	48. roof	73. comb	98. puff
24. Nero	49. rope	74. car	99. pipe (baby)
25. nail	50. lace (lass)	75. coal	100. disease

Notice that I've given you choices for a few of the numbers. Select whichever creates a stronger picture in your mind. Because, after a while, as you use the Peg Words, it will be that picture that comes to mind when you hear or see that number, not the word. When you hear or see 14, you'll immediately "see" a tire in your mind, *not the word "tire."* So, if you think you'll use Peg Words up to 100, learn those listed, or make up your own words, so long as they fit the Phonetic Alphabet and don't confuse with any of the other words. For example, *can* would be fine for 72, except if you're using a tin can for #12.

Throughout the years, people have asked me for a list of Peg Words up to 1,000. I've always discouraged learning so many Peg Words. It simply isn't necessary. It's better for you to think up a word or phrase for a 3-digit number when and if you need it. If you're faced with 942, it's easy enough—once you know the phonetic sounds—to arrive at *brain, brine,* or *prune.* Doing it that way is important for another reason—you're forced to concentrate on the number, to *think*, and as I mention often enough, that's important.

Now, on to bigger and better things!

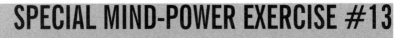

SPECIAL MIND-POWER EXERCISE #13

The coin problem we tackled in Chapter 12 reminded me of this somewhat easier-to-solve coin problem.

Lay out six coins like this:

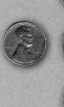

The mental exercise is to move only one coin so that you have four coins in each row—four in the horizontal row and four in the vertical row.

CHAPTER 14

Use It Or Lose It

"It is not enough to have a good mind.
The main thing is to use it well." —René Descartes

The "cliché" title of this chapter really fits when it comes to your memory, especially your memory after age fifty. What's important is to know *how* to use it. (I just saw a news piece on television about memory and older people. And this was the cliché the "professor" discussing this "scientific study" used about four times. What this twelve-week[!] study was all about was having older people use *rote memory* to try to learn poems and such. That's it and that's all! At the end of the study one elderly gentleman was asked if his memory was any better. His answer was, "Er, uh, well, gee, yeah, I think so.")

Please! Gimme a break! What a waste of time. Rote memory (defined in the dictionary as "a memorizing process using routine or repetition, often without full attention or comprehension") is on the same page with doing crossword puzzles. I think the people doing these kinds of studies should definitely read this book, don't you? For Pete's sake, I want to, and do, *eliminate* the need for most rote memory. I don't make you *use* rote memory. Forgive the redundancy, but—please!

Showing off what you've already learned is fine. There's nothing wrong with feeding your ego a bit and, more important, successfully executing a memory feat instills confidence and locks in the technique for you. So, having someone number a paper from 1 to 10, or 15, or 20 and remembering randomly called-out items by number is great for your self-esteem—but *most* important, you're using your memory

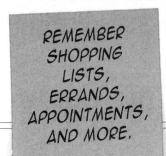

REMEMBER SHOPPING LISTS, ERRANDS, APPOINTMENTS, AND MORE.

in an appropriate way, a good way, a way that provides you the best mental/mind/memory exercise and keeps you sharp at any age.

Off to the Races

Each person, of course, has different memory needs, different "problems" to solve using my methods, strategies, and techniques. So it's difficult for me to select an "overall" example, a memory problem that *you* personally need to solve.

Years ago, the gentleman (call him John) who called the races at Yonkers Racetrack in New York had a *specific* memory problem. Say he was following the race through his binoculars and calling it, and the Number 6 horse started to take the lead. John had to look at his list of horses, to see the name of the 6 horse. By the time he looked up and started to say "Fast Arrow is taking the lead," Fast Arrow was no longer *in* the lead! John's problem, of course, was that he needed to be able to quickly memorize the numbers and names of the eight horses in any race. I taught him the Peg Word idea (visualizing a large shoe streaming though the air like a *fast arrow*) and—problem solved.

Ten by Number

In real life you don't usually receive information haphazardly, as when doing a memory feat. You usually receive information in order and memorize it that way. Let me try something with you. I'll give you ten items, corresponding to numbers 1 to 10. I want you to work with me and memorize the items as I've taught you to do. As usual, it's a good mind exercise, and there'll be a bit of a surprise afterward. So don't look ahead, keep your attention *here*, okay?

For #1, I'd like you to remember *church*. Form a ridiculous mental picture of *tie* and church. Perhaps, millions of neckties sitting in church, or you're wearing a church instead of a tie. See the picture.

#2 is *bear*. Associate/connect *Noah* and bear. You might see many bears boarding the ark two by two. Or, a large bear has a long white beard. Select one of these pictures, or one you thought of yourself, and see it in your mind.

#3 is *soldier*. Your *ma* is a soldier; see her marching or whatever comes to mind that a soldier does. I'm going to stop saying "See that picture" each time. I think you know that that's of utmost importance. If you don't "see" it there's no guarantee that it will come back to you.

#4 is *search*. You're searching for a bottle of *rye* whiskey or a loaf of *rye* bread. That could be too logical a picture, so be sure to make it ridiculous is some way. Finding *millions* of the item would do it for me.

#5 is *ledge*. You might see a cop (*law*) walking the beat on a high ledge, or a judge is on a high ledge banging his gavel.

Remember that when you have the time, it's not a bad idea to *review*. At this point, say the first five Peg Words to yourself and see if the item jumps to mind. That's the quick review.

#6 is *speed*. You can visualize a gigantic *shoe* moving at high speed. Remember that these are the silly pictures that come to *my* mind. Use whatever comes to yours.

#7 is *jury*. There are *cow*s sitting in all the seats of the jury box.

#8 is *bale*. Visualize a bale of *ivy*, or bales of hay are climbing up a wall like ivy.

#9 is *people*. Millions of *bee*s are stinging many people, or people are buzzing around like bees.

#10 is *power*. You can use lightning to represent power. If so, you can see lightning bolts shooting out from between your *toes*, or striking your toes. Or, mentally "connect" *power* drills to your toes.

You might want to review numbers 6 to 10, just as you did 1 to 5. That is, mentally count with Peg Words instead of numbers, and see if the items come to mind.

The Bill of Rights

If you know all of the items I gave you, what you've done, basically, is learn the Bill of Rights, the first ten Amendments to the Constitution! Keep in mind that I selected the one word from each that I knew would remind *me* of the complete thought, the amendment. You might very well select different words or phrases for the same purpose.

You may not care at all about knowing the Bill of Rights, but that's not the point. The point is to demonstrate that you can do it if you *want* to do it—no matter how old you are! You can learn and remember complex lists. The assumption in this case is that you are learning the Bill of Rights because you *want* to know it, so you are familiar with the ideas in it. If not, you could put more information into each of your associations. So…

1. Church—to remind you of "freedom of religion, press, speech." Obviously, you could have used *press* or *speech* as your reminder.

2. Bear—to remind you of "the right to *bear* arms." Different meanings, of course, but the *reminder* is there.

3. Soldier—to remind you of "freedom from quartering soldiers." *Quarter* would also remind you of the amendment. Remember that you can put more than one thought into any mental picture. In this case, *Ma* to *soldier* is fine, but you can get *quarter* into the same picture. (Your ma is a quarter and marching or fighting like a soldier.)

4. Search—to remind you of the "guarantee against unreasonable *search* and seizure." In my own original picture, I searched for the rye and *seized* it when I found it.

5. Ledge—I took some liberty here. I wanted to be reminded of privi*lege*, which reminds me of "privilege against self-incrimination." If you were doing this on your own, you might have chosen to see a cop arresting you (*law*), or you'd be in front of a judge "pleading the fifth."

6. Speed—to remind you of the "right to a speedy trial."

7. Jury—to remind you of "the right to trial by jury."

8. Bale—to remind you of "excessive *bail* and cruel and unusual punishment prohibited." Again, two different "bales," but still a reminder. A picture of gigantic *ivy* punishing someone would also have worked.

9. People—to remind you of "people's rights retained." You could have inserted "rights" (a prizefighter throwing rights) or "retained."

10. Power—to remind of "residual powers revert to the states."

You now know/remember the Bill of Rights, the first ten Amendments to the Constitution. Please understand that I've suggested words to include in the associations that I know would bring the entire thought, amendment, back to me. We are all individuals. If you really wanted to remember them, you would include what you knew would remind *you* of the entire thought. I've run through it with you as (a) an exercise and (b) to demonstrate how this aspect of my system can be used in a practical way. You may have a child, grandchild, niece, or nephew who'd love to learn how to do what you just did! (And apply the technique to other schoolwork.)

Shopping Lists

So many people have said to me, "Gee, I write things down and I still forget them." An interesting analogy is, "Gee, I wear a twenty-pound rock around my neck and I still can't swim well!" It's probably *because* you write things down that you don't remember them. They go from the source to the paper but they never go through your mind. You make no effort to remember them; you're *depending* on the paper rather than your memory. If you use the writing as an adjunct, as part of the remembering process, that's okay—but that's not usually the case.

"I write out my shopping list for the supermarket, then I forget to take it with me, forget to look at it, or lose it," is another complaint I've heard often. Yes, you can lose a piece of paper—but you can't lose your mind! (If you did, you wouldn't care too much about whether or not you remembered all the items, would you?)

It may not be an earth-shattering problem, but it can be a time-consuming and aggravating one. You don't want to come home after your shopping trip and, as you unpack your purchases, exclaim, "Oh, heck, I forgot the milk!" Back to the car, open the garage door, etc.…

Eliminate that pain in the neck. Form a Link of the items you need to buy. If you want to write them at the same time, fine, but many of my students have told me that they did that at first and soon realized that they never had to look at the written list—so they stopped making lists altogether.

Assume you want to buy milk. I haven't yet taught you how to remember the first item of a Link, just how to work backward from any Linked item. Well, it's easy: associate the first item with *yourself*. Or there's another way to do it. You now know something that represents #1, the first of anything: *tie*. So if you're starting your Link with *milk*, see a large container spilling its milk all over you, or see yourself wearing a container of milk around your neck instead of a tie. Use whichever you feel will work better for you.

Next, you know you need bread. Make *milk* remind you of *bread*. (Do not just visualize yourself having a slice of bread with a glass of milk. That's too logical an image, it isn't *ridiculous*; you'll forget it.)

Slap in the Face

I'm going to go off on a small tangent here to stress the importance of making your mental images ridiculous, silly, or impossible. You want to take them out of the ordinary, out of the mundane, because it is the everyday, ordinary, mundane things we tend to "forget." (I usually put quotes around "forget" to remind you that what I really mean is "don't remember in the first place.") You're not originally aware of the mundane, everyday things; they don't register in your mind in the first place. Ridiculous or silly things make an impression.

When one of the ancient philosophers was teaching a student and he made a statement that he deemed important, he slapped the student's face, hard. The idea was that the student would then never forget that statement! In the 1800s, when people were moving west and claiming land, a father would show his firstborn son where their property ended. And, as the boy looked, the father slapped him, hard. Again, the assumption was that the "slappee" would never forget where his property ended.

The problem is that slapping hurts! I prefer to do it mentally. The slap was meant to focus attention. A *ridiculous* mental image does exactly the same thing, it focuses attention—*but without pain.* It's my *Slap-in-the-Face* Principle. Again, the idea isn't new. This comes from a parchment more than two thousand years old, called *Rhetorica ad Herennium*: "When we see things that are petty, ordinary, and banal, we generally fail to remember them because the *mind isn't being stirred by anything novel or marvelous.* Ordinary things easily slip from the memory while the striking and the novel stay longer in the mind." (The italics are mine.)

Of course. For thousands of years no one paid attention to this simple idea. I did!

Back to Shopping

All right, you've associated milk to yourself and now you need milk to remind you of bread. Perhaps a slice of bread is drinking milk; that's ridiculous. Or, you're pouring slices of bread out of a milk container. Next, you need dog food. Make bread remind you of that. Visualize walking a large slice of bread instead of a dog (the bread is doing what a dog does when you walk it). Then make dog remind you of oranges: you're walking a gigantic orange like a dog, or a dog is peeling and eating a large orange. Your next picture might be you, peeling an orange and there's a head of lettuce inside. If you feel you need a better reminder for lettuce, use "let us." And so on. You can make the Link as long as necessary. Since each "image" is a separate one, the number of items doesn't matter; one leads you to the next. That's the point.

When you're in the market, you don't need to get the items in the sequence of the Link. That might involve too much back-and-forth with the shopping cart (which is okay if you want some physical exercise along with the mental exercise!). Just go over your Link mentally and pick up the items you need as you go through the store. Whatever is nearby, throw into your cart. Keep going over your Link and anything you haven't yet put in the cart will stand out in your mind so you can go and get it. To be sure you have everything, go over your Link as you approach the checkout counter—that's your final reminder.

Try it. What have you got to lose?

Errands/Appointments

You can apply exactly the same idea to remembering your errands and appointments. Take, for example, flowers to postage stamps to key to ice-cream cone to umbrella to cash to nails to book.

Gigantic stamps are growing like flowers; you're using a gigantic stamp instead of a key to open your door, or you're putting a large key on an envelope instead of a stamp; you're licking a large key instead of an ice-cream cone or a gigantic key is eating an ice-cream cone; you're holding a dripping ice-cream cone over your head like an umbrella (in the rain), or an ice-cream cone is walking in the rain carrying an open umbrella; you open an umbrella and cash (millions of bills) falls out of it, or you're paying for something with umbrellas instead of cash; you're hammering cash (bills) into something instead of nails, or you're paying with lots of nails instead of cash; you're hammering nails into a gigantic book or you open a book and millions of nails fly out and hit you in the face, or a gigantic nail is reading a book—and so on.

There's your errand/appointment list for tomorrow. You need to stop at the florist, you have to go to the post office for stamps, you need to have a key made, you have to remember to call Mr. Cohen, pick up an umbrella, stop at the bank for cash, pick up nails, and pick up that book you promised to get for your spouse. You can form the Link the night before. In the morning, while brushing your teeth or at breakfast, go over it. If you've left something out, add it onto your Link then. It takes no extra time away from your busy schedule.

Again, the errands need not be done in order; the point of using a basic Link is to remember (and accomplish) everything before you pick up your car or board the train for home. Of course if you'd rather remember them in numerical order, you can associate your shopping list or list of errands to your Peg Words. Perhaps that would work better for you.

I'll be talking to you later about remembering things to do at specific times—like when to take certain medications. Right now, think about what you've learned in this chapter. I'll continue to show you how to twist and manipulate the basic ideas I've outlined so far, to solve any memory problem.

You ain't seen nothin' yet!

SPECIAL MIND-POWER EXERCISE #14

Imagine this: You're faced with three boxes, each containing two marbles. In one box are two white marbles. The second box contains two black marbles, and the third box holds one black and one white marble.

The boxes are labeled *WW*, *BB*, and *BW* (white/white, black/black, black/white).

The problem is, some joker has switched those labels so that *each box is INCORRECTLY labeled*. You want to restore order, so that each box is labeled properly again. You may remove one marble at a time from any box without looking inside the box. Remember—only *one* marble at a time.

Your mind-power question is: What is the *least number* of marble removals you can do to accomplish this?

CHAPTER 15

Real "E State"

"The memory strengthens as you lay burdens on it, and becomes trustworthy as you trust it." —Thomas DeQuincy

I taught you how to remember the first ten amendments to the Constitution mainly as a mental exercise, but if knowing/learning/remembering all twenty-five amendments is important to you for any reason, memorize them all by doing as you've already learned. Select a word or phrase from each amendment, a word or phrase that you know will bring the entire amendment to mind; then associate that word or phrase with the vital Peg Word. Memorizing the amendments from 11 to 25 will continue to add to your brain power, besides adding a few more pieces of information to your already vast "knowledge fund." Ready? Here are the rest of the amendments:

11 – Exemption of states from suit

12 – Method of electing president and vice president

13 – Slavery abolished

14 – Protection of citizens' rights

15 – Right to vote

16 – Income tax (easy to form a ridiculous picture here!)

17 – Election of senators

18 – Prohibition

19 – Women's suffrage

20 – Abolishes the "lame-duck" Congress

21 – Repeal of Prohibition (hic!)

22 – Limits president's terms in office

23 – Residents of District of Columbia given vote in presidential elections

24 – Poll tax abolished

25 – Presidential disability and succession

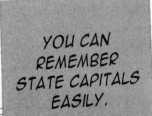

YOU CAN REMEMBER STATE CAPITALS EASILY.

If you do try to memorize all the amendments, the strategy of selecting one word or phrase to bring a complete thought to mind will become even clearer to you, as will the use of Peg Words in conjunction with the Substitute Word/Thought technique.

State Capitals

In the preface of this book I mentioned a few of the questions that Mrs. Goldfisher asked on her tests in grade school. One of those questions was, "What's the capital of Maryland?" What I didn't mention in the preface is how I manipulated the tiny bit I'd learned from old books on memory training in order to remember the capitals of *all* the states. (There were only forty-eight of them then.) I was sure that Mrs. Goldfisher would be asking for capitals of other states on future tests. What I did for Maryland was to visualize *an apple is land*ing on *Mary*'s head. *Mary land* = *an apple is* (for Annapolis).

I did that kind of association with every state, moving alphabetically from Arizona to Wyoming. What's interesting is that by the time I finished associating "shy Ann" (Cheyenne) to a large letter *Y* roaming (Wyoming), I knew most of the state capitals *without* thinking of my mental connections, because—and I know I'm repeating myself, but it warrants repetition—I had, without realizing it and without pain, concentrated on each as I never could have before, *in order to* come up with the association. But the ridiculous pictures locked 'em all in.

To this day, I do a "state" demonstration at some of my appearances. The audience members each have a numbered list of the states in alphabetical order, along with their capital cities *and* their populations. Someone calls out a number from 1 to 50, or a capital, or the name of the state itself, or its population, and I immediately give the rest of the information. I won't go into the populations here, but if that interests you, you already know how to handle long-digit numbers. As one example, in my original "picture" I associated *moon* (32nd state, alphabetically) with *new cork* (New York) and *all bend knee* (Albany) and *dove tips cars* (18,190,740, the population of New York at that time).

Learning just the states and their capitals is easy and is a wonderful over-fifty mind exercise. I've listed them all here for you, along with my suggestions for a Substitute Word or Thought. As usual, you can use those or come up with your own Substitute Word or Thought. I've numbered the states, but whether you want to remember them by number is up to you. I'll leave it to you to create the mental image, the ridiculous picture, which includes all of the information that you want to associate with each state. Here's an example of how I would proceed: For 24, I'd see a married woman playing the fiddle (Nero) as she sips liquid (Mrs. Sip) and a *jack* operated by her *son* is lifting her up. (The 24th state is Mississippi, the capital is Jackson.)

1 (tie) Alabama/Montgomery – alley bum, or album; General Montgomery (the beret he always wore), or mount gum airy.

2 (Noah) Alaska/Juneau – I'll ask her, or baked Alaska; d'you know? Or June, oh.

3 (ma) Arizona/Phoenix – air zone; fee nix, or Phoenix rising.

4 (rye) Arkansas/Little Rock – ark and saw, ark can saw, ark Ann saw; little rock.

5 (law) California/Sacramento – call a fawn (yeah); sacrament or sack men toe.

6 (shoe) Colorado/Denver – color a doe (or toe); den where?

7 (cow) Connecticut/Hartford – connect a cut; hard Ford or hard fought

8 (ivy) Delaware/Dover – Della wear, tell her where; dough for, dove

9 (bee) Florida/Tallahassee – flower there; tall lass see

10 (toes) Georgia/Atlanta – George, gorgeous; hat lander

11 (tide) Hawaii/Honolulu – how are ya', ha why E; honor Lulu

12 (tin) Idaho/Boise – Ida hoe, potato; boy see, noisy

13 (tomb) Illinois/Springfield – ill noise; spring field

14 (tire) Indiana/Indianapolis – indian; indian nap (pole is)

15 (tail) Iowa/Des Moines – I owe her; the mine, day mine

16 (dish) Kansas/Topeka – cans ass, can sass; toe peeker, the peeker

17 (dog) Kentucky/Frankfort – can't talk, Ken tuck E; frankfurter

18 (dove) Louisiana/Baton Rouge – Louise see Anna; baton rouge (red)

19 (tub) Maine/Augusta – (horse's) mane; gust (of wind); august

20 (nose) Maryland/Annapolis – Mary land; an apple is

21 (net) Massachusetts/Boston – mass chew sits; boss ton

22 (nun) Michigan/Lansing – mix again; land sing

23 (name) Minnesota/Saint Paul - mini soda; t'aint Paul (or pull), sand Paul

24 (Nero) Mississippi/Jackson – Mrs. sip; jack son

25 (nail) Missouri/Jefferson City – misery, miss airy; d'ya have a son, chef a son

26 (notch) Montana/Helena – man tan her; Helen, hell and her

27 (neck) Nebraska/Lincoln – new brass car; Lincoln penny (or car), link on

28 (knife) Nevada/Carson City – never there; car son (city – see tea, sit E)

29 (knob) New Hampshire/Concord – new hemp (or ham) sheer; con (prisoner) cord

30 (mouse) New Jersey/Trenton – new jersey (cow); train ton

31 (mat) New Mexico/Santa Fe – new sombrero, new mix a coat; Santa (fee)

32 (moon) New York/Albany – new cork; all bend knee, all ban E

33 (mummy) North Carolina/Raleigh – I use "wind" to remind of "North"; wind carry liner; raw lea, roll E

34 (mower) North Dakota/Bismarck – (wind) decoder, the coat; bees mark

35 (mule) Ohio/Columbus – oh, hi O, high O; Christopher, call him boss

36 (match) Oklahoma/Oklahoma City - OK homer; OK homer, see tea

37 (mug) Oregon/Salem – ore gone; sail M, sale ham

38 (movie) Pennsylvania/Harrisburg – pen sill vein; hair is berg, Harry's berg

39 (mop) Rhode Island/Providence – rode island; prove dance, provide Ns

40 (rose) South Carolina/Columbia – sows carry liner; column bee

41 (rod) South Dakota/Pierre – sows decoder, sow the coat; pier

42 (rain) Tennessee/Nashville – ten I see, tennis E; gnash villa

43 (ram) Texas/Austin – taxes; awes tin

44 (rower) Utah/Salt Lake City – you tar, ewe tar; salt lake (see tea)

45 (roll) Vermont/Montpelier – vermin; mount peeler

46 (roach) Virginia/Richmond – virgin, where gin; rich man, rich mount

47 (rock) Washington/Olympia – washing ton; oh limp (pier)

48 (roof) West Virginia/Charleston – vest virgin; the dance, Charles ton

49 (rope) Wisconsin/Madison – wise con sin; mad at son, medicine

50 (lace) Wyoming/Cheyenne – Y roaming; shy Ann

Do it, form your mental images. Not only will you amaze yourself but you'll have developed a large number of new brain cells! In forming your mental pictures, you can visualize people you know, such as George for Georgia, Helen for Helena—you get the idea.

SPECIAL MIND-POWER EXERCISE #15

You'll build up lots of valuable brain cells trying to come up with the solution to this one.

Think of a word to which you can add *one* syllable and make it shorter.

That's it!

CHAPTER 16

Important Numbers

"Thinking is the hardest work there is, which is the probable reason why so few engage in it." —Henry Ford

I've taken you away from long numbers for a couple of chapters just to give your mind a bit of a rest, not that it really needs it. I've talked about remembering things (Bill of Rights, states and state capitals) that may not be of importance to you, although they're certainly important for exercising your mind, for building those brain cells and "training your brain," Now, let's zero in on a few ideas that you will use in real life.

Telephone Numbers

Richard Himber was a well-known musician; he was also a magician, which is how we originally met. We became close friends. I mention him here because he was the first person I know of who made it easy to remember his telephone number by having it match his name. When you dialed "RHimber," you reached Richard. As you probably remember, in the early 1960s telephone numbers included exchange names such as OXford, STerling, ESplanade, PEnnsylvania, BUtterfield, and RHeingold.

You dialed the first two letters of the exchange, then five digits, as in BU 8-1234. Himber's exchange was *RH*eingold, which is what gave him the idea. His number was RH 4-6237: RHimber! Nowadays, it's not uncommon for people or businesses

CULTIVATING YOUR "IMAGINUITY."

to associate words with their phone numbers. (I'm sure you've seen the ads for 1-800-DIVORCE, and the like.)

And now, of course, you can put telephone numbers into the "memory" of your cell or landline telephone. This is probably the main reason that telephone numbers are "forgotten": once they're in your phone's memory, you never think of them again.

Many people tell me that it is still a pain in the neck not to remember telephone numbers, as it sure would be for me, particularly when I'm calling information for a number while in my car, where no paper or pencil is handy.

Avoid the "pain" by utilizing what you now know: the Phonetic Alphabet and the Substitute Word strategies. We no longer need to remember exchange names—but now we have three-digit area codes with which to contend. Simply connect your words for the complete number, including area code, and use a Substitute Word or phrase for the person's or company's name!

Let's first discuss the numbers without the area codes. Mr. Walker's number is 746-9021. What could be easier now? Just "see" yourself (or anyone) walking—you're a *walker*—and you *crash* (746) into a *peasant* (9021), or perhaps *poisoned* came to mind. And, if you have to, if the number is told to you quickly, use your up-to-99 Peg Words. But it's knowing the *sounds* well that's key.

Now, if Mr. Walker's area code is 314, add *motor* or *meter* to your mental image. After using the same word for the same area code a couple of times, you'll develop standards for area codes: *butter* or *batter* for 914; *mats, moats,* or *meats* for 310; *no tune, not me,* or *need him* for 213; *church* or *George/Georgia* for 646; *buttock* or *paddock* for 917; *Indian, antenna,* or *nothin'* for 212; *latch* for 516 (see next paragraph); *nest* for 201; *pest* for 901, *bottom* for 913; *mask* for 307; *miser* for 304; *retire, rotor,* or *reader* for 414; *rotten* for 412; and so on. If it's an area code you haven't heard before, just make up a word for it and that's what will come to mind the next time you hear that area code.

Yes, I know, *latch* really transposes to 56, not 516, because you don't pronounce it "latitch." But, since I know the context in which I'm using the word, I simply *know* that it means 516 *in this context:* it has become my "standard." Similarly, I can use *in'* instead of *ing* (as in *nothin'*) because I *know* that I'm doing so. I also know that it couldn't be "nothing" because that transposes to four digits, and area codes all consist of three digits. This is a good example of how to make the strategies work for *you*.

So, Mr. Smith's telephone number is 201-648-9470: See yourself smashing a *nest* with a large black*smith*'s hammer; a *sheriff breaks* the hammer, or arrests you.

Dr. Ames's number is 715-410-2009. See yourself *aim*ing (Ames) a stethoscope (doctor) at *cattle* (715; or you could use *cuddle*). Connect that to *rats* and *noses up* (all the rats put their noses up), or to *nice sip* or *news soap*.

Jab long ski might be your Substitute phrase to remind you of Mr. Jablonski. Your original mental image might have been that you're jabbing a long ski as it floats in a *channel* (or the ski is made of *chenille*) that's full of *papers* (or party *poopers*, or *paupers*). Do that, and you know that Mr. Jablonski's number is 625-9940 (channel papers). Include a word for the area code (perhaps *fuses* for 800) if you want to. You don't necessarily have to break a telephone number into three- or four-digit groups. Use whatever comes to mind, so long as it fits phonetically. *Chain ill baby rose* would also tell you Mr. Jablonski's telephone number.

If you'd like to have your electrician's number at your fingertips and his number is 862-9421, you might "see" an *electric* plug *fishin'* (862) and drinking *brandy* (9421); or visualize *fashion brand*.

Extension, Please

If you need to remember intercom or extension numbers, the same strategy applies. One corporation executive said to me, "Harry, please teach me and my people how to remember those damn intercom numbers. That'd save us lots of man hours and the stiff necks caused by looking from the phone to the paper where those numbers are listed."

Just apply the strategy; it's so simple. Miss Ross's extension is 116. Associate either *to touch, to attach, dotage,* or *tot itch* to *roars* or *rose.* Mr. Leventhal's extension is 101. Connect *test* or *toast* to *eleven tall, leavin' tall,* or *vent tall.* Mr. Byrnes's intercom is 121. Associate *burns* to *tent* and you'll never forget it. The shipping department's extension is 712. Visualize lots of *cotton* being *shipped.*

I could give you a bunch of telephone numbers with which to practice, but if you really want "practice," start *applying* the strategy to real numbers in your life. That'll do it. Using my systems is the best practice of all. They are the only skill I know of that you can start to use immediately. The "practice" is in the doing.

Zip Codes and Addresses

People in the mail-order business, or in any business that involves lots of mailing, know that being familiar with zip codes saves lots of time, as does remembering complete addresses. Associate *man hat* (Manhattan) to *disease* and you'll know that most Manhattan (NY) zip codes start with 100.

If you need to remember that Mr. Knapp's address is 946 West 95th Street, NYC 10025, form your mental picture. Perhaps you're napping (Knapp; if you want to remember his first name, Bill, a gigantic bill is napping) on a porch (946) wearing a 10-gallon hat (my standard picture for "west"; you can use *vest* or *best.* I use *yeast* or *beast* to represent "east"). The hat is made of *new cork* (New York, or use the Empire State Building). The cork is ringing a large *bell* (95th Street) as that bell *tosses a nail* (10025; or use *disease nail*). You can visualize this in a second, certainly in less time than it took me to write it all out. Prove it to yourself—just try it.

Here are a few suggestions for some zip codes: 30264 – mason chair, mouse nature; 07450 – score lass, scare less, squirrels; 90715 – basket low, pass cattle; 10014 – tosses tire, dozes there, ties stare; 11978 – tote up coffee, tot pick off; 10016 – teases dish; 90402 – pass raisin, buys raisin; 10128 – taste knife; 95742 –black rain, plaque run; 30374 – mouse maker; 89014 – ivy paster (or poster, pastor).

Prices

No need for me to take up much space to tell you about remembering prices. You already have all the "equipment" you need to be able to do so. Well, all right, I'll use a bit of space because I want to give you some mental exercise. I'll make up some prices of specific items and then you can take a short test to see how you're doing.

Toaster – $49.15. Connect toaster to *reptile* (perhaps you're toasting reptiles, or a toaster is slithering around like a snake). Obviously, you know that the toaster you're interested in doesn't cost $4,915.00! So reptile can only mean $49.15. But, in circumstances where you do want to "break it down," use a different word or phrase to tell you the dollars in front of the decimal point and another word for the amount, the cents, after the decimal point. For $49.15, *rope tail* or *rob towel* would do it. Be sure to "see" the picture of toaster to reptile.

Camera – $315.95. You're entering a gigantic camera, it's a *motel* (315), or you're taking many pictures of *metal* as a *bell* (95) rings. Use whatever you think of, but *see* the picture.

Chair – $147.10. Chair to *targets* or to *trick toes, truck toes.* Select one, and see it clearly.

Car – $18,995.00. A *dove* is driving a *car* and teaching a *pupil* (to drive). You could use *dive pupil, tough pupil, dove babble.* Select one, etc.

You might want to do a quick review of the first four items and their prices at this point.

Lamp – $71.50. Lamp to *cute lass* or *cutlass.* Form your mental image and really *see* it.

Cell phone – $59.50. Cell phone to *lapels, labels, lip lass, lap lace.* Select one and make your association.

Pen – $21.75. Pen to *nautical* or *neat coal.* See the picture you've selected.

Computer – $1,750.00. Computer to *tickles, tackles, talk less, tie calls.* This is the last one, so be sure to see the picture your imagination has helped you create.

Review, if you like, then fill in the blanks:

Lamp $ _____   Computer $ _____

Camera $ _____   Chair $ _____

Car $ _____   Pen $ _____

Toaster $_____   Cell phone $ _____

See what I mean?

Stock Prices

The only difference here is the fact that there are usually fractions involved. The strategy I teach is to make up a word to represent the dollars, a word whose last consonant sound tells you the *eighths.* Simply change all fractions to eighths: ¼ is two eighths, ½ is four eighths, ¾ is six eighths. Then connect your word/picture to the name of the stock.

For a stock selling at 49½, you might use *roper.* The last consonant sound tells you "four eighths," the *rp* of "rope" tells you the dollars, 49. Now, if you're wondering why *roper* won't remind you of 494 (no fraction) for the associated stock, you really shouldn't be buying and selling stocks! You certainly should know if you paid in the $49 range or the $494 range for a stock. And if a stock is 494½, you could use *repairer.* Do you see why?

So, *racket* will represent, remind you of, 47⅛; *friar* 84½ (four eighths), and so on. Then you can simply associate the "price word or phrase" to your representative picture of the stock: *telephone* for AT&T, for example; *Mack roar E* for McCrory Corporation; *Polar herd* for Polaroid; a *mini soda* for Minnesota Mining; a car saluting a general for General Motors, and so forth.

A single mental image of a *Mack* truck *roar*ing at an *E* (or an *eel*) that's squatting on a *melon* would remind you that McCrory is selling at 35¼ (*melon* = 35 and two eighths).

Stock symbols are made up of letters of the alphabet. I haven't yet discussed how to make letters of the alphabet *tangible*, visual in the mind. I will do that soon, and then we'll talk about stock symbols.

A Piece of Pi

This falls into the category of Not Important Numbers. Recently, there has been interest in memorizing pi up to hundreds and thousands of decimal places, and I have gotten e-mails from people telling me that they've used my system to do just that. One person writes that in just about three weeks he's already memorized up to 10,000 places; his goal is 50,000 places! Well, to each his own. If you want the mental exercise, here are the first few dozen digits of pi:

3.1415926535897932384626433832795028841971693993751058209

You might start your long Link like this: Motor, tulip, angel, my love, pick up, man (or main) mover, chain, charm, move mink up, lesson, fiver, topic, touch up, mop up, my colts, lovin' (or leaven, leavin') speaker...

As usual, these are the first words or phrases that came to my mind. You may have thought of and Linked motor, tail pinch, all my love, pick up my name, virgin (or freshen), charm, move mink, blessin' (or pulls in, pale sun, pleasin'), fevered, pick up chip, mop up, Michael (or mogul), tussle, fins up, car...

If you want to go further, look up more places and then "do" as many digits as you like each day. Review each time before continuing the Link.

This has been a very full chapter, so take a break and go over the "stuff" you've learned.

Now, I want to talk just a bit more about

Interest, Creativity, and "Imaginuity"

I talked about the importance of interest in memory in chapter 6 but I need to mention it again. Sure, what we refer to as "memory" may get less and less reliable as we age. I know that when I'm not applying my systems, I sometimes fumble over words and familiar things may fall into that "senior moment" abyss. But that never happens with any information, any word, any name, any number, any *anything* that I'm *interested* in. That's my point.

As we grow older, it's *possible* that our mental faculties decline a bit, but our interest in things *definitely* does. We simply aren't as interested in certain things as we were when we were younger. And because we're not as interested, we don't *listen* as closely, as intently, as carefully, as we used to. Perhaps we don't *care* as much. I don't know if you can teach old dogs new tricks, but I *do* know that I can teach "old people" new tricks—as I'm doing right here, right now.

Applying my memory-training methods *forces* interest; you *have to* listen, focus your attention, in order to apply those methods. I'll tell you what else goes along with the application of the systems: as you apply them you are automatically exercising your *imagination* and your *creativity*. To form the crazy/ridiculous associations, the mental images, you must use your "imaginuity." That's a word "marriage" I made up, the marriage of imagination and ingenuity, both essential parts of creativity.

Remember: *using is exercising*. Of course it's important to exercise your imagination. According to Henry J. Taylor, "Imagination lit every lamp in this country, produced every article we use, built every church, made every discovery, performed every act of kindness and progress, created more and better things for more people. It is the priceless ingredient for a better day."

It's your imagination—exaggerating sizes and amounts, using one thing instead of another—that aids in forming those crazy and *memorable* mental pictures and associations. If you laugh to yourself at some of the images you come up with, that's good. *Fantasize.* Albert Einstein said, "The gift of fantasy has meant more to me than my talent for absorbing positive knowledge."

Okay. I just wanted to assure you that there's method to my madness—in addition to the fact that there's a bit of madness to my method!

SPECIAL MIND-POWER EXERCISE #16

There is a common eight-letter English word that contains only *one* vowel; it is also one of our longest one-syllable words.

Trying to come up with that word is a strong mental exercise.

Remember, it is a one-syllable word that's eight letters in length and contains only one vowel.

If you don't want a hint, don't look below.

Hint: There are two hints in the way I've worded the exercise.

CHAPTER 17

Send Me a Telegram

"No matter how abstract or intangible information is, I'll show you how to make it 'stract' and tangible." —Harry Lorayne

I have a feeling that this chapter won't make it into the book, so I'm probably writing it just for myself! I think my publisher and editor will feel that there aren't very many people interested in learning and memorizing the Morse code, so it's silly to take up valuable space with it. (To tell you the truth, I'm not even sure the Morse code is still used.) What I hope they'll realize is that it's one *heck* of a mind exercise. Part of what you'll learn here will come in handy for other memory problems, such as the stock symbols I've previously mentioned, and what's more, learning the Morse code demonstrates how my systems can be manipulated, altered, or twisted to solve *any* memory problem. Besides...I want to teach it to you because I'm awfully proud of it!

First, a short anecdote. When I was in the army (that's World War II, folks, not the Civil War!) and training in the infantry, the colonel in charge heard about me. (I'd been showing some of my memory stuff to my bunkmates.) One afternoon he made a quick remark to me about it. Now, I'd been told that the men in the Signal Corps were required to take a six-month course: three months to learn/memorize the Morse code symbols (the dots and dashes) and three months to practice the tactile stuff on the key, the sending and receiving.

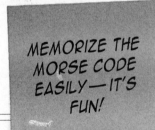

MEMORIZE THE MORSE CODE EASILY— IT'S FUN!

Since I was young, naive, and brash, I blurted out to the colonel, "You know, sir, I can teach the men in the Signal Corps the Morse code symbols in an hour or two." Inwardly, I was thinking, "Wow, a chance to do some good. I can save the country all those man hours—and maybe even get out of some of the infantry training!." The colonel looked at me, eyebrows raised, and exclaimed, "Are you nuts?! Then what the hell would we do with them for the three months?!"

"Of course, sir," I said. And I never saw him again.

Alphabet Words

I can and do teach people the Morse code dots and dashes in an hour or so. The first thing you need to do is learn a word that represents each letter of the alphabet. That shouldn't be hard for you now. You'll know them, basically, after reading them once. What I've done is use a word that *sounds like* the letter. Like this:

A	*ape*, *hay*	N	*hen*, *enema*
B	*bean*, *beet*	O	*old*, *eau* (water), *owe*
C	*sea*	P	*pea*, *peek*
D	*dean*, deal	Q	*cue* (stick), *queue*
E	*eel*, *eek* (scream)	R	*hour*, *art*, *argue*, *aardvark*
F	*eff*ort, ha*lf*	S	S curve, *ass*, *escape*
G	*gee*, *jeans*	T	*tea*, *tee*, *T*-square
H	*age*, *itch*, *ache*	U	*ewe*, *you*, *eunuch*
I	*eye*, *I*	V	*veal*, *V* for victory
J	*jay* walking, *Jake*, jail	W	Waterloo, trouble you
K	*cake*, *cane*, key	X	*eggs*, *X*-ray
L	*elf*, *el*(elevated) train, he*ll*	Y	*wine*, *wild*
M	*hem*, *ham*, *emperor*	Z	*zebra*

I use *bean* for the letter B because *bee* would conflict with the Peg Word for #9. For W, I "see" Napoleon; for R (hour), I see a clock. So you see, even the abstract symbols that are the letters of the alphabet *can* be visualized. But wait—I know that dots and dashes (·−) are even more abstract and less meaningful to you. How on earth can they be pictured or visualized? Well, this is what I'm so pleased with. I have arbitrarily assigned the letter R to all dots, and the letter T or D to all dashes. That solves the problem!

Once you set that concept in your mind, that only the letters R and T (or D) have meaning here, you're halfway to *easily* learning the Morse Code symbols. All you have to do is use a word or phrase that can be visualized and that contains Rs and Ts in the *proper sequence*, and connect it to the vital letter of the alphabet.

Here's what I mean. There's really no way to visualize the Morse code symbol for A (.–), not when there are twenty-five other combinations of dot/dash symbols. But it's easy to visualize a *rat*! And, in my system, *rat* can represent *only* .–: there's an R and a T, in that order, in that word. Now you can form a ridiculous association of the two visual entities, the letter A and its "code word," *ape*, and *rat*. A = . –!

I still get a thrill teaching this, I really do! And, if you don't want to bother with the letter words (ape, bean, sea, etc.), when I'm through teaching this method, I'll teach you another way that you might find easier or like better. Right now, if you want the mental exercise, associate ape to rat, bean to terror, C to torture, and so on.

A	·–	rat		**N**	–·	tier (door, deer)
B	–···	terror		**O**	–––	touted (deeded, taught it)
C	–·–·	torture		**P**	·––·	rotator (rudder, red door)
D	–··	tearer		**Q**	––·–	tethered (tied right)
E	·	air (eerie)		**R**	·–·	writer (reader, red hair, rotor)
F	··–·	rear tire (rare tar)		**S**	···	error (roarer, rarer)
G	––·	tighter (tidier)		**T**	–	toe
H	····	rarer rye (or ear)		**U**	··–	rarity
I	··	rower		**V**	···–	re-arrest (airier route)
J	·–––	ratted		**W**	·––	retied (rated, raided)
K	–·–	trout		**X**	–··–	turret
L	·–··	retire her (restorer)		**Y**	–·––	treated
M	––	tot (toad; tight)		**Z**	––··	teeterer

I've given you choices for some letters; obviously you'll want to use the one that you can visualize more clearly. You know what to do now: associate the two important entities. For J, perhaps you see someone jay-walking and you *ratted* on him, or you're in jail because someone *ratted* you out. I visualize Napoleon, with his hand between the buttons of his jacket, for W (Waterloo), and I see myself tying him up. The ropes are loose, so I *retied* him. See yourself making an *eff*ort to change your *rear tire*; a gigantic clock (*hour* for R) is a *writer*, and so on.

Another Method

The other method I mentioned is my "adjective" strategy. You use the "code" words (for the dots and dashes) but not the alphabet words (for the letters). Instead, use an *adjective* that begins with the vital letter. *A*wful rat, *Big* (or *Bad*) terror, *C*ruel torture, *D*umb tearer, *E*xcellent air, *F*lat rear tire, *G*irdle tighter, *H*ot rarer rye, *I*diot rower, all the way to e*X*cellent turret, *Y*ou treated, *Z*igzag (or *Z*any) teeterer.

Of course, you can make up your own adjectives to place before the code words, making sure that they begin with the appropriate letter of the alphabet.

What do you know? I guess I convinced my editor that learning the Morse code might be useful after all.

SPECIAL MIND-POWER EXERCISE #17

In this store, 1 costs 10 cents, 43 cost 20 cents, 123 cost 30 cents.

Can you explain this? Can you figure out what I am buying?

This is *not* a trick question.

If you don't want a hint, do *not* look below.

Hint: I am in a hardware store.

CHAPTER 18

Stock Market Symbols

"Harry, I've developed a tremendous amount of ability by using your memory systems to remember things that would otherwise have taken me many years to learn. I now learn very quickly. Memory has a great deal to do with furthering knowledge." —Vic Sperandeo

In his book *Trader Vic: Methods of a Wall Street Master* (John Wiley & Sons, Inc., 1991), Vic Sperandeo tells how he "aced" an interview for his first job in finance. He won out over a couple hundred other young people because he used my memory techniques to remember *every* stock symbol of that time—more than *sixteen hundred* company names and their two- or three-letter symbols!

Just as the interviewer was about to end their discussion ("Don't call us, we'll call you"), Vic blurted out that he'd memorized all of the stock market names and symbols. The executive insisted that that'd be impossible, and he started to test Vic—who, of course, answered all of the questions without even one mistake. He was hired on the spot!

Vic is a fan of mine. (Hey, I can use all the fans I can get!) In his book, he says, "Harry Lorayne dramatically influenced my life, he was a role model…," and more. I blush—but I'm so pleased that

he went on to become "Trader Vic," a very successful "Wall Street Pro," using my systems all the while in both his work and his personal life.

TRIUMPH OVER THE TICKER.

I may not be able to help you become

that successful in the stock market, but I can certainly help you remember company names and their stock symbols. (I've already taught you how to "do" company names and prices.)

You surely don't want to remember *all* of the symbols, as Vic Sperandeo did, but you can easily remember the few you need or want to. It's easy because you already know how to visualize a company name and you also know how to visualize letters of the alphabet (as you learned when I taught you how to remember the dots and dashes of the Morse code). I told you there'd be other uses for the technique.

For some symbols, you won't need the alphabet words. For example, the symbol for Pittway Corporation is PRY. All you have to do is visualize a gigantic *pit pry*ing its way out of something. That does it; you have the reminder of the two entities—*pit* for Pittway and *pry* for PRY. If you'd rather, you could use alphabet words to "connect" *pit* (and how much it *weigh*s) to *pea* (P), clock (hour, or R), and *wine* (Y): PRY.

The symbol for **Boeing** is **BA**. See someone bowing (either bending at the waist or using a bow and arrow!) as *beans* (B) are being thrown at him by an *ape* (A). There are always choices—you can visualize someone bowing as he receives his BA degree, or bowing as someone says, "Bah." If you were really trying to remember these things, you'd automatically lock in the first image that comes to mind.

The symbol for **Marion Labs** is **MKC**. I'd see a dress (*hem*, M) *marryin'* in a *lab*oratory. It holds up a wedding *cake* (K) and throws it into the *sea* (C). If you can visualize a girl named Marion, that will do, too, as will dogs (Labradors) for Labs.

Shaw Industries is **SHX**. You might imagine millions of *eggs* (X) coming up on a *shore* and you "Sh" them (sh *eggs*) for SHX. An *ass* (S) scratching an *itch* (H) with an *exit* (X) sign would also do, as would "*shucks*," if that came to mind.

Polaroid is **PRD**. *Prod* a camera, or *prod* a *polar* bear; or you can associate *pea, hour, dean* to camera or polar bear. (A million peas fly out of a clock and hit a dean; you take a picture of it with your Polaroid camera.)

Philip Morris, Inc. is **MO**. Your *ma* (or *Moe*, the diminutive for Morris) is throwing a dress (hem/M) into water (*eau* /O). If you think it's necessary, get *full lip* or *fill lip* (Philip) into your silly picture.

Polymer Corporation is **PLM**. Seeing a *polly* (parrot) being a *ma* (polly ma = Polymer) to a *plum* (PLM) would do it, as would a silly picture of *polly ma* to *pea hell hem*.

Borden, Inc. is **BN**. You *bought* a *den* full of *beans* and *hens* (BN), or connect *bought den* to *bin*. Just a *ban* on milk (reminds me of Borden) would do it for me.

Newmont Mining is **NEM**. Visualize a *hen* (N) and an *eel* (E) eating a *ham* (M) on a *new mount*ain, and you've got it.

The mental images I suggest, or those you think of yourself, are like instant mental calisthenics: it just takes longer than an instant for me to write them. And forgive the repetition but, again, half the battle is won even before you actually *see* the picture because you've pinpointed your concentration, focused your attention on the memory problem as you never were able to do before.

Bear in mind that you can put whatever you want to, any information, into one mental image. If you want to remember the company, its stock symbol, *and* its current price, simply include your word for the price in your picture. So, if Polaroid is selling for, say, $175, get *tickle* or *tackle* into your company-to-symbol picture. If the price is 175½, and that "half" is important, "tackle*r*" or "tickle*r*" does it: that translates as 175 and four-eighths.

Again, I know I won't make you a "Wall Street Master," but by using my systems, you will surely be able to remember stock symbols and prices better than you ever did before.

SPECIAL MIND-POWER EXERCISE #18

Think about this one for a while.

See if you can place five odd digits—single digits, that is—into a basic addition problem whose total is an even number.

No tricks, no double meanings.

It's a good mental exercise.

CHAPTER 19

One-Upmanship

"Instant erudition...how to be marvelously, maddeningly, devastatingly, engagingly impressive about art, literature... without actually knowing all that much about them."

The above was part of the advertising for a series of booklets titled *The Bluffer's Guide*, back in 1971. Aside from art and literature, the series covered music, cinema, opera, and wine, with facts about each category that allowed a person to "follow in the delightful tradition of one-upmanship."

Each booklet was introduced by David Frost—and that's how I got into the picture. David was a fan, and had an Emmy-winning television talk show on which I appeared quite often. Of course, he knew of my expertise, so, to encourage sales of the booklets, he enlisted my help.

It was the sheer quantity of facts in *The Bluffer's Guide* that created the problem. You couldn't carry a booklet around with you all the time—you had to *memorize* the facts! David asked me to choose one of the subjects, memorize all the facts about it, then appear on his show as an "expert" in that subject, just to show that it could be done. I chose *wine* as my category, probably because I knew less about it than I did about any of the others. I memorized all the facts in *The Bluffer's Guide to Wine* and David promised that he'd ask only about things that appeared in it. He would also have a real wine expert on the show with me.

REMEMBER FACTS AND SHOW OFF YOUR CULTURE QUOTIENT.

Long story short—I held my own and the wine expert oohed and aahed at my knowledge. We had him fooled. Then a wine table was wheeled onto the set for a wine *tasting*. I hadn't been told about this, and I really didn't know how to "taste." I particularly didn't know that you were supposed to take a sip, swish it around in your mouth, then spit it out. (*That's* what that bucket was for!)

Well, I tasted, *swallowed*, tasted some more, swallowed some more, as I spoke about the "cru" and the different vineyards, and so forth. (Boy, was I winging it!) And by the sixth or seventh "taste" I was slurring my words! Guests have appeared on shows already drunk, but I think I have the distinction of being the only one ever to get drunk *on the show*!

I think the wine specialist figured out that I wasn't such an expert after all—but I knew more than enough facts to fool him and the rest of the world. It was great for sales of *The Bluffer's Guide*!

You needn't try to remember all (or any) of the information that follows—unless you want to. I'm not going to test you on any of it. What I'm interested in here, as you should be, is the concept, the idea, the method, the way to apply the system to learning facts about any subject. Please, come along with me.

Literature

It's easy to remember facts, trivia, if you will, on any subject. Charles Dickens wrote *A Tale of Two Cities*. The first thing that comes to my mind as I start to memorize that fact is a gigantic *tail* with *two cities* on it, and they quarrel (or there are *quarrels* = Charles) like the *dickens*! Here are some more.

Rabbit Run – **John Updike.** See a *rabbit run*ning *up* a *dike*— what could be easier?—and you've locked in the two entities, title and author. I'm sure you can get a *john* into your mental image if you feel the need for it.

Dangling Man – **Saul Bellow.** You're *bellow*ing at a *dangling man*. "Sole" or "soul" in the picture would remind you of Saul.

Naked Lunch – **William Burroughs.** Visualize a *burro* and a *naked* person eating *lunch*. Or, there's a naked person eating lunch in all five boroughs of New York City.

The Waste Land – **T. S. Eliot.** There are lots of cups of *tea* (T) and lots of *ess* curves (S) in *a lot* (Eliot). It's *a lot* of *wasteland*. Again, keep in mind that I always suggest the first image that comes to my mind. You may want to try to think of your own. You might have thought of seeing millions of tea bags as you exclaim, "Tea's (T. S.) *a lot* (Eliot), or use *L E yacht*.

East of Eden – **John Steinbeck.** See *yeast* in the Garden of *Eden*; there's also a large beer stein there, which you take back: *stein back* (Steinbeck), *yeast in Eden* (*East of Eden*).

The Invisible Man – **Ralph Ellison.** Usually, all you need in your picture is the author's last name but as you know, you can include whatever you like. You can "see" a large, *rough* (Ralph) letter L being your son (L is son – Ellison) and it is fading, becoming *invisible*.

Lord of the Flies – **William Golding.** Visualize a gigantic fly as it *lords* it over all the other *flies*; he writes his *will* on a *yam* with *gold ink* (will yam, gold ink).

The Magic Barrel – **Bernard Malamud.** Imagine a *barrel* doing *magic* tricks. See it start to *burn hard* (Bernard) so you *mail a mud* (Malamud) pile to it to put out the fire.

Ulysses – **James Joyce.** *You list Es* as someone *aims* (James) *juice* (or *joys*) at you.

The Catcher in the Rye – **J. D. Salinger.** You're in *jail* (J) with a college *dean* (D) and you both are watching a baseball *catcher* waist deep in *rye* (*Catcher in the Rye*) whiskey because he injured the *sail* (*sail injure* = Salinger) of his boat.

Alcestis – **Euripides.** "Connect" *you rip Ds* (or *Europe a tease*) to *Al says this*.

Of course, you can include any facts that you think are important into any association. For example, if you want to remember that Sidney Carton is one of the main characters in *A Tale of Two Cities*, as is Madame Defarge, you can get *sit knee carton* and an elegant lady (or whatever "Madame" conjures up in your mind) eats *the fudge* into your picture. Please understand that the sounds needn't

141

be exact—true memory will tell you the correct pronunciation. All you need is a *reminder*. *The barge* will remind you of Defarge if *you* make the small effort to think of it.

The setting of *Alcestis* is outside the palace at Pherae. Include in your picture of *you rip Ds/Al says this* a *fairy* or *ferry* (outside a palace). It's all up to you.

Art

Many teachers have attended my memory seminars and it never fails that one of them exclaims, "Why, oh why, don't we teach this in school?" Good question.

The artist **Mondrian** was a constructivist; one of his paintings is called *Broadway Boogie-Woogie*. See a *man dryin'* a huge *construction* site. See the drying man dancing the boogie-woogie on Broadway (a broad way, or a wide street with lots of lights), and you'll remember the artist, his style, and the painting.

Who painted *The Birth of Venus*? **Botticelli** did. A *bottle* and a *cello* (or *bought a cello* or *jelly*) get together and give birth to an *armless woman* (most people associate this with Venus, although she doesn't appear armless in Botticelli's painting) or *V nuts*. *Botticelli* also painted *The Calumny of Apelles*. *Column knee* and *apples* in your picture would be a reminder.

A couple of **Henri de Toulouse-Lautrec** posters are *La Goulue* and *Jane Avril*. *Low track* (Lautrec) to *la glue* and *chain off reel* would remind you of that. If you want, you can include *too loose* for Toulouse and/ or *awn real* for Henri.

See a *van go* to *seize Anne* (**Van Gogh, Cézanne**) so that she can make impressions on a post (they are postimpressionists). *Says Anne* would also do as the Substitute Thought for Cézanne.

Salvador Dali is a surrealist. See a *doll* that's *sure real*. See that "sure real" doll sitting on a *flying* horse (*Pegasus, or peg asses, peg aces, peg is us, pea gay sauce*) to remember that he painted *Pegasus in Flight*. If you need to, get *salve a door* into your picture to remind you of Salvador.

142

To remember that **Rauschenberg** is considered a pop artist see a *roach* on an ice*berg* drinking *pop*.

Monet was an impressionist. *Money* (or *moan eh* or *A*) *impresses*.

El Greco's real name was Kyriakos Theotokopoulos. Want to remember that, so that you can show off your knowledge? Well, one way would be to associate *L crack O* (El Greco) to *carry our coats* (Kyriakos) to *the O to cop, alas* (Theotokopoulos). *The O to cop, alas* (say it rapidly) will remind you of that ordinarily hard-to-pronounce (much less, remember) name.

Ma sell to *the champ* (or *do charm*) will remind you of **Marcel Duchamp**. See *the champ* take off all his (or her) clothes and descend a staircase to remind you that Duchamp painted *Nude Descending a Staircase*.

One of **Picasso**'s many paintings is the mural *Guernica*. *Pea car so* (or *sew*) connected to either *g'way knicker* or *go wear knicker* would lock in that fact for you.

A *ram brand*ing a human reminds that **Rembrandt** was a humanist. See the branding going on at *night* as many *watch* to remind you that one of Rembrandt's famous works is *Night Watch*. That painting hangs in the Rijksmuseum in Amsterdam, where I stared at it for a long time. "Rikes museum" is the closest I can get to the pronunciation. The R is rrrolled, and if you get *rakes museum* into your picture (you see the rakes and exclaim "*yikes*") I'll wager that you'll remember it *if*, in fact, you *want* to remember it.

Edvard Munch (pronounced "muhnk") was an expressionist. You're *express*ing yourself to a *monk*. Visualize the monk emitting a horrible *scream* and you'll remember that Munch painted *The Scream*, one of my favorite paintings. It's in the Munch Museum in Oslo, Norway. (*Ah, slow, no way*).

Can you imagine *Sir Rat* (or *sewer rat*)? Then you've got **Seurat**. See him pointing at everything (Pointilism) on a Sunday afternoon. See it being done on an island when you hear a *grand shot* (or *jot*). You can see Sir Rat *gorg*ing himself (for George). Georges Seurat invented the technique known as Pointilism. His most famous painting (and another of my favorites) is *Sunday Afternoon on the Island of La Grande Jatte*.

Music

Haydn composed the "Sunrise Quartet." Visualize a sunrise as a string quartet plays; you're watching the sunrise from your *hay*-filled *den*.

Verdi wrote the opera *Falstaff*. You're asking a *staff* "Where D?" and the staff *falls*. If you get *eye E there* or *I eat here* into the picture, you'll know that he also wrote *Aida*.

Associate *strive and ski* or *straw wins key* with *pet rush* (or *roach*) *car* to help you remember that **Stravinsky** composed *Petrouchka*. Get a *bird* on *fire* and *write off spring* into your association and you'll know that he also composed *Firebird* and *Rite of Spring*.

Rose in knee (**Rossini**) being trimmed by a *barber* who is *civil* (just "barber" should suffice) tells you that Rossini wrote *The Barber of Seville*.

Just a small point, here. I've been to Seville, Spain. Something happened to me there that will always be fresh in my mind and will always remind me of Seville, so, that's what I would picture here. I mention it because I want you to keep in mind that your Substitute Thought can be *anything*—so long as it reminds you of the desired thing. That's why, as I've already mentioned, the older you are, the more knowledge and experience you have, the more "weapons" you have to help you visualize things (or people or whatever you wish). This is one of the ways that getting older means getting better!

Back to Rossini: Connect *rose knee* to a *large O* (or *ahh, go*) on a *totem* pole to help you remember that he also wrote "Largo al Factotum."

Moe's art connected to *marriage of figs* in *a row* reminds that **Mozart** wrote *The Marriage of Figaro*. Include an image of a flute doing magic and you'll know that he wrote *The Magic Flute*.

Debussy composed *La Mer*. Associate a large letter *D* being *bossy* (D bossy = Debussy) to a *llama* or use *the sea*, if you know that "la mer" means "the sea" in French.

Tchaikovsky wrote *Swan Lake* and *Sleeping Beauty*. Visualize a *shy cow ski*ing near a lot of *swans* on a *lake*. See one swan who is a *beauty sleeping* (*The Sleeping Beauty*).

Wagner wrote *Lohengrin*. Associate *wag knee* (or *wagon, ah*) to *low an' grin* or *low N grin*, to lock it into your memory.

Cinema

The very first Academy Awards ceremony was held in 1928, for films produced between August 1927 and August 1928. Best Actor was Emil Jannings; Best Actress was Janet Gaynor. The Best Movie was *Wings* and Best Director was Frank Borzage (pronounced "bore-zay-gee"; hard *g*). If you'd like to memorize this information you can start a link with *knife* (28) or *tub knife* (1928). To that, "connect" *a meal* (Emil) *jan*itor *inks* (Jannings) to *Jan*uary, or to a girl named Janet if you know one whom you can visualize; *chin net* would also do, to *gain oar* (Janet Gaynor) to *wings*, to a *frank*furter to *boar say key*. Perhaps, a gigantic *knife* is eating *a meal* as a *jan*itor pours *inks* into the food; the inks freeze because it's *Jan*uary and very cold. You *gain* a large *oar* to protect you from the cold; the oar sprouts *wings*, eats a *frank*furter—shows some frankfurters to a *boar* (or *bore*) and says, "If you want some, *say key*."

The images I suggest are just that: suggestions. Use them or come up with your own. Either way, you are giving your imagination one hell of a workout.

See yourself *brand*ing an *O* (Brando) on a *coin* ('72) and you'll know that Marlon Brando won Best Actor in 1972. *Lies a man, Ellie* (or *L E*) will get you to Liza Minelli, who won the prize that year for Best Actress. That same year, *The Godfather* was the Best Movie and *bob fussy*, also associated to "coin" tells you that Bob Fosse was Best Director.

Imagine Clark Gable (if you can picture him; if not, use *clock able*) using a lawn *mower* (34) to tell you that Mr. Gable won Best Actor in 1934. Include a *cold beer* (or *cold bear*, Colbert) in that picture to tell you that Claudette (*clawed hat*) Colbert won for best actress that year. See it all *happening one night* and get a *cap* cheering "*rah*" into the picture and you'll know that Best Movie and Best Director that year were *It Happened One Night* and Frank Capra.

So, you see? You really can remember any kind of trivia, in any category, this way. Staying with "cinema," if you want to remember all, or most, of the movies directed by, say, Billy Wilder, you start a Link. Start with *wilder*, then you might see yourself going wild (or wilder) in an apartment (*The Apartment*) in which it gets very hot, but *Some Like It Hot*. Someone eats a gigantic fortune cookie in the hot apartment (*The Fortune Cookie*), and so on.

It's easy to associate a movie title to a director if, for some reason, you want to impress with that knowledge. For example, see *the seeker* or *D seeker* (Vittorio De Sica) seeking the person who stole his bicycle (*The Bicycle Thief*) and you've got it. If you want to, get *V tore E O* for Vittorio, into your picture.

Wine

One of the things (among quite a few others) that I did for my "wine expert" appearance on *The David Frost Show* was to memorize the glossary at the back of *The Bluffer's Guide to Wine*. Being able to nod knowingly, or to respond when an "in" word was mentioned, and to drop "in" words myself, really added to the illusion. To do this, I connected words to meanings just as I taught you to do for foreign language vocabulary and unfamiliar English words.

Aigre refers to the sourness caused by acetic acid. I visualized myself holding my nose because of a sour smell while standing in a large *acre* of land. I got "I see Dick" into the picture for "acetic" acid.

Brut means "very dry." Connect *brute* to *dry*.

Cru means "growth." I visualized a *crew* growing. The *r* is a back-of-the-throat sound.

For **Foudres**, associate *food ray* to a large capacity vat in which wine blending is done.

The word **marc** refers to a liqueur made from the last pressing of grapes. I saw myself *mark*ing only last pressings.

I associated *moose sew* to *sparkling* so that I could remember that **mousseux** means just that: sparkling.

Vin de pays refers to "peasant" wine, as does **vin ordinaire**. A picture of *van pay* to *peasant* is all I needed.

Punt is the term for the hollow found in the bottom of certain wine bottles. *Punt*ing a football that hits the bottom of a gigantic bottle causing a hollow does it.

Sec means "dry." *Sack* to *dry*.

Sir ah to *black grape* told me that the word **Syrah** referred to a species of black grape found in the Rhône Valley. I simply put *rowin'* (for Rhône) into my picture.

And, just for good measure, I Linked the five principle producers of Médoc. I Linked *medic* to *ma go* (**Margaux**) to *can't enact* (**Cantenac**) to *paw E yak* (**Pauillac**) to *sand jewel E N* (**Saint-Julien**) to *saint S step* (**Saint-Estèphe**).

I'm getting a bit high just thinking of all those "wine" words—and thinking about how easily you, too, can become an overnight know-it-all!

SPECIAL MIND-POWER EXERCISE #19

This will take a bit of thinking and experimenting. That, as you know by now, is the point. The thinking and experimenting, the trying to work it out, is the mental exercise.

Okay, then:

> **Chickens cost 50 cents each**
> **Ducks cost $3.00 each**
> **Turkeys cost $10.00 each**

The problem is: You want to buy *exactly* 100 of the birds and spend *exactly* $100. How many of each should you buy?

CHAPTER 20

Computer Tutor

"All knowledge is but remembrance." —Plato

Many mature people are starting to get involved with computers. I'm one of them. I held off for years. My earlier books were written in longhand and then on typewriters, starting with the old mechanical Royal.

Well, I finally let myself get talked into acquiring a computer. It's most likely my dyslexia, but I found, and still find, computers difficult to understand. A friend, a computer "maven," was trying to teach me some computer stuff. I interrupted, and said, "Hey, slow down, plain English, please; pretend I'm ten years old." He answered, "Harry, if you were ten years old I wouldn't have to be teaching you—you'd be teaching me!"

It's we older people who need all the help we can get. Now, please understand, I can't help you *understand computers*. What I can and will do is help you in the "remembering" area—because there is a lot to remember when learning how to use a computer. The frustration is in trying to retain specific information. In my case, that would be something like how to tell the machine to leave my e-mail messages on the server so that I can access them later, from a different computer. It's awfully tiring, boring, time-consuming, and damn annoying to keep looking that up "somewhere."

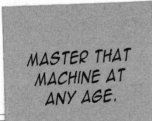

MASTER THAT
MACHINE AT
ANY AGE.

And what in the world do all those "F" keys across the top of my keyboard mean? What are they for? What does Ctrl/Alt/Delete do for me, and how do I remember it? I need to remember the functions of Ctrl/E, Ctrl/L, Ctrl + Shift + A, et al.

Well, let's talk about it. I won't talk to you as if you're a ten-year-old, but I'll use the KISS idea: Keep It Simple, Stupid! Do you know why? Well, I've told you why…because I don't understand most of it myself—but I can remember every bit of it that I *want* to.

It's important for me to stress that the specific things I'll talk about apply only to the specific computer I'm familiar with. Remember that I'm teaching you an *idea* and I have to use examples. If those examples don't apply to *your* computer, *change them accordingly.* If you don't, they may confuse you or cause harm, and I certainly don't want that on my conscience. Are you with me? Let's barge ahead.

A great help to me was to memorize "navigational sequences." (I think that's the terminology!) Because they *are* sequences, you can apply the Link system to them—so the first thing you have to do is to create a Substitute Word or Thought for units of the sequence. You'll need an image for Tools, Options, Accounts, and so on. I'll mention the images I use as I come to each one in the examples that follow.

I have computers in two different locations and each one uses Outlook Express 6. I need my e-mail messages to appear on both of them. So, I had to "do" this sequence: Tools/Accounts/Mail/ Properties/Advanced, then click on "Leave a copy of messages on server." (That's the sequence for *my* computer; you will have to check the specifics for *yours*.)

To remember the sequence, start with a "heading" that tells you where you want to go, the *result* of the actions. For this example, "messages on server," your "heading" ridiculous picture might be of a *server* (a butler or waiter) with messages or telegrams all over him. Start your Link from that. Visualize *tools* (screwdrivers, hammers, wrenches—that's my standard image for "tools") all over him; then connect "tools" to "accounts." Since these are actions that come up often, I use a standard image for each. For "accounts" I see a man in knee breeches, wearing a monocle: *a count.*

I "see" tools hammering, etc., on *a count.* I want accounts to lead me to *mail,* so a count is covered with or surrounded by mail. Mail has to lead to "properties," for which my standard image is many small houses. So I visualize millions of pieces of mail streaming out of each of many houses (properties).

My picture for *advanced* is of soldiers advancing from out of the houses. When I click on "advanced" the screen I need appears, and I check the box next to "Leave a copy of messages on server."

It just took me three paragraphs to explain it, but actually forming the Link of *tools* to *accounts* to *mail* to *properties* to *advanced* (usually written Tools/Accounts/Mail/Properties/Advanced) takes a matter of seconds. If your computer uses the latest (at this writing) Vista system, the sequence is a bit different. It's tools/accounts/ your email address/properties/advanced. That sequence will lead you to the box you need to check. Decide on Substitute Words or Thoughts and form your Link.

If I want to tell my computer to remove e-mails from my server when I permanently delete them (so that they don't pile up and clog the server) I go through the same sequence, because that option is there to be checked or unchecked on the same final screen. But if you're using Outlook 2003, then the sequence is Tools/Email Accounts/Next/Change/More Settings/Advanced.

For "next" I use *necks* or I see myself on a line waiting to be called "next." For "change" I see *coins.* For "more settings" I might see myself sitting over and over again because "more sittings" reminds me of *more settings.* (You could use *moss ate things.*) Once you decide on your Substitute Words or Thoughts, simply form your Link. That leads you to the window or screen in which you can check the proper option.

Also in Outlook 2003, if you want to change the size and font of the e-mails on your screen, you have to go to Tools/Options/Mail Format/Fonts. Decide on an image for "options" (I see people selling options on the floor of the stock exchange). *Shuns* or *up chins* would also do; remember, it's what *you* think of that works best. For "format" try *floor mat*; "fonts," *founts.* Again, once you have your representative images it's easy to form your Link. Remember always to start your Link with the "result" you're aiming for. In this case, I'd start with a *fount* that grows and shrinks continually, to remind me of *font* and *size.*

To do the same thing in Outlook Express 6, it's Tools/Options/ Compose/Font Setting: an almost instant Link. I don't think I have to tell you the image I use to remind me of "compose," but I will—a *composer* working at his piano. What else? (If you are using Vista, it may be create mail/format/font/make your selection/OK.)

In Outlook 2003, if you'd like to have your signature (and/or your address, even your picture) automatically added to every e-mail, you'd go to Tools/Options/Mail Format/Signatures/New. For "new" I always see the item it's being connected to as *shiny and sparkling*.

All right. You've got the idea and, to repeat, it's the *idea,* the strategy, that's important. Who knows? When you're reading this the examples I've selected may be obsolete. It doesn't matter. You'll always need to form a Link to remember the navigational sequence to a "result." Now you know how to do that.

More Computer Tips

Do you want to put an acute accent mark over a letter, like this: é? On my computer, when I'm in Word (it doesn't work when I'm sending an e-mail), I have to press Ctrl + ' (apostrophe) and then the letter. I think of *a cute* girl (you can imagine her speaking with an *accent*, if you think it necessary; I don't) *pass*ing a *trophy*. "Control" is a key you'll use often so create a standard in your mind for it. I use a *roll*. You can visualize yourself not being able to roll something; *can't roll* = control. A *can troll*ing (for fish) would also do. For this purpose, associate *a cute* girl *control*ling how you *pass* a *trophy*.

For an "accent grave" (è) press Ctrl + ` (the accent grave symbol—it's the key way at upper left on my keyboard). For a caret (ê) over a letter, press Ctrl + Shift + ^ (it's on the 6 key) then the letter. Can you see yourself *shift*ing something as your Substitute Thought for the Shift key? Or, visualize a shifty character. *Roll* to *shifty* to *carrot* does it for me. One more: if you want an umlaut or prickar over a letter (ë), press Ctrl and Shift and then : (colon). Again, Link *roll* to *shifty* to umlaut (*I'm loud, some lout*).

You can use your "alphabet" words to good advantage here. In e-mail, Ctrl S saves a letter to your "Draft" folder. (*Roll* around an *ess* curve in a *draft*.) Ctrl A highlights everything in a Word document or an e-mail message, so *roll* an *ape* under *high lights*. (Click once on the screen to get rid of the highlighting.) Ctrl Z corrects your last mistake. Ctrl X *cuts*, Ctrl C *copies,* Ctrl V *pastes.* Form your own quick, simple reminders.

Visualize *roll*ing an *eel* to *center* and you've "locked in" the fact that Ctrl E starts your typing (in Word) at the center of the page. *Roll* an *elf* to the left—Ctrl L—gets you back to "align left," typing from left of the page. Ctrl + Shift + A is an "All Caps" command: *roll* a *shifty ape* near the *cap*itol building.

My standard image for the Alt key is an obvious one, *halt*. You can see yourself erasing something to represent "delete." If you press the Ctrl/Alt/Delete keys all at the same time, it will bring up the Task Manager in Windows. See if you can form a quick Link to lock this information into your mind. (On most computers, pressing Alt and F4 at the same time clears your screen. See yourself *halting* (Alt) *fur* (F4) and the fur disappears or clears.)

Decoding Air France

Years ago, an Air France employee showed me a booklet she'd received from the main office. It was about "Francis," the airline's computer system. The booklet, *Aide Memoire* (aid to memory) purportedly helped employees remember the computer system's codes. Actually, all it did was *list* the codes; no memory aids were included. The Air France employee, along with some colleagues, came to me for "memory aids." Most of the codes were letters—no numbers involved. All that was needed was my strategy for visualizing letters of the alphabet and forming ridiculous mind images.

At that time, the code for "available seats" was FG. Just "seeing" a *fig* searching for an available seat would do it; so would imagining gigantic figs seated in all available seats. And, of course, associating *half* (F) *jeans* (G) to available seats served the same purpose.

Many of the simpler codes began with the letter W or D. WR stood for "search." I instructed them to visualize themselves *search*ing for someone or something during a *war*. WI was the format code for "print." *Why* would remind them of WI, so would *Waterloo* and *eye*. They could associate *print* to either of these Substitute Thoughts.

A series of D codes had to do with "cancellation of groups." Once in that format, a single letter told the reason for the cancellation. Just a D meant "could not confirm space." I told them to see a *dean* trying to attain space on a flight but no one would confirm it for him. N stood for "insufficient number of participants." I would see a *hen* looking for participants but it can't find enough. F meant "competition offered a better fare." *Half* (F) *fare* would do it (or *half* a county *fair*).

An Air France employee called a month later to tell me how grateful she was. She said she used the associations, and after the third or fourth time she simply *knew* the codes. That's the *point*.

Oh, she also used the "alphabet" idea to remember (and not have to look up) the three-letter codes for airports. Some are easy because the letters are an abbreviation of the city, like ATL for Atlanta and BOS for Boston. (To remember that it's Logan Airport in Boston, connect *low can* to *boss ton*.) But for New Orleans, it's MSY. She associated MiSsY to *oar leans* (or *hem, ess* curve, *wine* to *oar leans*).

FCO is Fiumicino Airport in Rome, Italy. *Half sea owe* to *roam* tells you that airport code; *fume see no* would help you remember the airport name. An *oar land*ing on an MC (master of ceremonies) who shouts "*Oh!*" reminds you that MCO is the Orlando, Florida, airport code; *me coy* tells you that it's McCoy Airport.

The same methods, using the alphabet idea and the alphabet words, can be applied whenever it's necessary to remember letters.

Cell Madness

I believe it was Clarence Darrow who said that with each bit of progress "we take a step or two backward." If he didn't say it, I'm saying it.

In the play, *Inherit the Wind*, the Darrow character points out that when the telephone was invented we gave up part of our privacy.

Of course. And with the advent of cell phones, we've given up more than just privacy. Now, we have to hear loud annoying rings and voices in restaurants, theaters, banks, post offices, everywhere. People using cell phones on the street walk right into you and then tell *you* to watch where you're walking. Holding the phone to their ears and talking while driving—well, I don't think I need to express my opinion about that!

Cell phones are like mini-computers now, so I need to devote a sentence or two to them. I recently succumbed. On my telephone I need to press "star"/86 to get my messages. To remember this I immediately made an association: I visualize a *starfish* coming out of my cell phone with messages all over it. Star/*fish*—perfect. I never have to think about it again. If it were star/28, you could see a knife (28) shining in the sky like a star; get *messages* into the picture.

To increase the volume of my ring tone, I press star/18—so I "see" a dove (18) shining in the sky like a *star* and making louder and louder noise.

To update or program my cell phone, I dial star/228. Again, I imagine a *star* dropping its knife— it has *no* k*nife* (228), and it's creating a *program* to procure another one. As usual, that's what *I* used; make up your own association, of course. Star/646 tells me how many minutes I've used. *Star church* associated with *used minutes* takes care of that.

If I want to see my own cell phone number, I press Recall (RCL) then pound (#). To lock this in my memory, I see myself trying to *recall* my number in vain. I *pound* the phone in frustration. Or you could get "weighing a *pound*" into your picture.

I see myself *functioning* quite well around an *ivy*-covered wall and I start (or the ivy starts) to *vibrate* in order to help me remember that I have to press FCN (function) and then 8 in order to change from ring mode to vibrate mode.

Well, you get the idea. Remember that these are the codes on my particular cell phone. You need to apply the concept to your own cell phone codes. On my phone, when I want to check whether I have Data Capability I have to press FCN, then 125. My original association was of half (F, for *F*unction) a grapefruit (my "standard" for *half*) going through a *tunnel*. You can decide to always start a Function image with the letter F. Then your picture might be *f*oot *n*ail, or *f*at *n*ail (F125).

Committing to memory the two-digit numbers for speed dialing is a great convenience and timesaver. When I need to call my garage, I know to press 12-Send because I originally visualized a large sheet of *tin* driving around in my garage. That's all. If I need to call my office, I press 22-Send; I originally "saw" a *nun* sitting at the office's front desk. My association of a large *sock* being a *rob*ber tells me that my son Robert's speed-dial code is 07-Send. To call my friend Gerald at home, I press 30-Send. I saw many *mice* running around his house. I didn't have to, but getting *chair* (or *share*) *old* into the picture got his name into the association as well.

There are more than eighty telephone numbers in my phone's memory and I never have to scroll through to dial any of them. All I have to do is connect the two-digit speed-dial number to the person's name, company name, restaurant name, as just taught.

There are times when I need to punch in a PIN code. I'm sure you do, too. You can make up a word for any PIN by using the Phonetic Alphabet and then connecting the word to your cell phone, bank, burglar alarm—whatever.

What's the Password?

Sometimes you need to know both a PIN *and* a password (or just a password). It's easy enough to remember both—as well as what the password is for.

When I want to start up my computer I need to type in a password. I'm not going to tell you what my real password is, of course! I'll just make one up for teaching purposes. Let's make the password *applepie*. Simply see yourself reaching into the computer to pull out an apple pie. Just "pie" would suffice.

Perhaps your password is *center*. See yourself pushing your hand through the *center* of your computer screen. You see? All you need to do is make the *computer itself* remind you of the password—until it becomes knowledge.

The password you need to do your banking might be *underwear.* See yourself depositing a pile of *underwear* instead of checks or cash.

F Is for Function

Finally, how about those F keys I mentioned at the top of this chapter? Honestly, I don't much bother with them, but that's not the point. I want you to know how to do it when and if you want to. Make up a word to represent each F key. Easy enough. Start each word with the letter F and make the next consonant sound represent the number. Check 'em out.

F1	fit or fat	**F5**	foil or foal	**F9**	fib or fop
F2	fan or fun	**F6**	fish or fetch	**F10**	fuse, fuss, or face
F3	fame or foam	**F7**	fake	**F11**	faded
F4	fire or fur	**F8**	five (-dollar bill)	**F12**	fatten or fit in

Each of the suggested words can be visualized and, as you certainly know by now, that's *key*. For F8 you can use *fever* or *favor*, if you'd rather. Do you see why? You know that there are only twelve F keys so you couldn't have a word for F14. You'd know that within this context, for this specific memory problem, *fever* or *favor* could only represent F8. I just wanted you to be aware of this idea. (Not all of the F keys have a function, not on my computer anyway—or, if they do, I don't know it!)

Press **F1** and a "help" screen pops up. This is handy. Visualize a screen or window so *fat* that it needs *help*.

F2 is used to rename an item or move text. Associating it with *fan* or *fun* would do it.

F3 opens a "find files" screen. Visualize yourself "finding files," which gives you *fame*.

F4 brings up your addresses, so maybe all of your addresses are on *fire*.

F5 is the "refresh" key. Scraping yourself with *foil* is refreshing; it makes you say, "Aah."

F6 moves your cursor around a program. Obvious, right? A *fish* swims around a program.

F7 has no functionality in Windows.

F8 accesses Safe Mode. Your *fever* isn't high, you're *safe*.

F9 has no functionality in Windows. (It may have in some individual programs.)

F10 activates the "menu bar" in many programs. A *fuse* reads a *menu* (at a *bar*, if you like).

F11 brings you to full-screen mode when working in Internet Explorer. Your *full screen* is *faded*.

F12 has no functionality.

Different activities are called into play when pressing Shift or Ctrl plus an F key. If you're interested, you can try them on your computer. Press Shift and the F7 key, and an English thesaurus appears on screen. Associate *shifty, fake*, and English (or *they saw us*). Ctrl plus F7 moves your document. You *roll* a *fake, moving* it (or *roll* in the *fog*). According to how you're visualizing "roll," you can see yourself eating a *fake roll*. Ctrl plus F10 maximizes the document. You're *roll*ing a *fuse* and it keeps growing (maximizing). There are plenty of others that I won't bother listing. Again, I just wanted to give you the idea.

Just a few more F's

Talking about all those Fs reminds me of an extra little mind exercise. Read the following and count the number of F's it contains.

FINISHED FILES ARE THE RE-
SULT OF YEARS OF SCIENTIF-
IC STUDY COMBINED WITH THE
EXPERIENCE OF MANY YEARS.

SPECIAL MIND-POWER EXERCISE #20

You can lay out five items, such as playing cards, in many different sequences. For example: 54321, 12345, 53214, 31452, 52314, etc.

Can you find a fairly easy way to figure out exactly how many different sequences are possible for five items? For seven items?

CHAPTER 21

It's About Time

A man's real possession is his memory. In nothing else is he rich,
in nothing else is he poor. —Alexander Smith

Did you remember to take your Lipitor today? Or was it four hours later when you smacked your forehead and exclaimed, "Darn it—the Lipitor!"? How about your Altace, aspirin, or Micardis? Wouldn't it be great if there was a pill you could take to help you remember when to take the pills you need to take every day, every week, or every month? Well, as I said in an early chapter, right now, *I'm* that pill!

If you have to take the same pill three or four times a day, it's easy enough to spread it out and remember to take them. Just take one at breakfast, one at lunch, one at dinner (and one before bedtime, if it is four times a day). Easy. But what if the schedule is a little more complicated? The simplest way to set up a schedule is to make your Peg Words represent hours of the day. What an interesting idea! I'll talk about a more direct and specific method later, but this may work fine for you right now.

It doesn't make sense to mentally go through your Peg Words starting with *tie* (1), because that'd be starting with one o'clock in the afternoon. Let's assume that you're up and functioning at 8:00 A.M. Start your mental countdown with *ivy* (8), and then let each Peg Word represent its hour. You can mentally go over the words *ivy, bee, toes, tide, tin* to bring you to 12 noon. For the afternoon, continue through *tie* (for 1:00 P.M.), *Noah, ma, rye, law, shoe,* and *cow,* which brings you to 7:00 P.M. (Since there is no zero o'clock, the *s* sound in *toes* represents 10:00.)

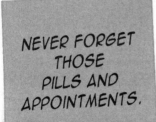

NEVER FORGET
THOSE
PILLS AND
APPOINTMENTS.

Now, you might think that using *ivy, bee*, etc., again, for the evening hours, will be confusing. I assure you that it won't be. True memory will tell you the difference—and besides, you probably know which medicines you take during the day and which in the evening.

But, if you want to, you can use different words/images that fit the system for 8:00 P.M. to 12:00 midnight. For example, *foe, boy* (or *buy, bay, boo*), *tease* (or *dice*), *tot* (or *tote, toad*), *tine* (or *dine*). Another way, of course, would be to use a 24-hour clock—but that really isn't necessary.

Okay, now you can visualize each hour of your day. So what? So you can associate the medicine you want to remember to take with that "certain hour"!

Let's say you take Lipitor every evening at about 9:00 P.M. If you're using your basic Peg Word, see a *bee* tearing your lip: *lip tore*. If you're using the secondary Peg Word that tells you that it is P.M., not A.M., visualize a *boy* tearing his lip.

How often you mentally go over your Peg Words is up to you, and depends on how many different pills you regularly take. Even going over them every hour or so is easy, because you can do it while doing any other physical thing, such as brushing your teeth, showering, having a cup of coffee, eating, and so forth. And there's some serendipity here: you're exercising your mind at the same time; you're keeping yourself *aware and alert*!

Each time you think *bee* or *boy*, you'll be reminded about your Lipitor. If it's Zocor you take, associate *sew core* or *soak oar* to your "hour word." Say you want to take Micardis every morning at 10:00 A.M. Think "*My card* is between my *toes*." See the silly picture. If you take aspirin (*ass pourin'* or *S peer in*) at 12:00 noon (*tin*), simply connect those two entities.

As I've already mentioned, you'll know which medications you take during the A.M hours and which during the P.M. hours, but you can always make things more specific if you want to. In this case, just put "*aim*" into your picture to represent A.M. or "*poem*" to represent P.M. (For example, you are *aim*ing a rifle.) You really need to use only one. That is, if you have *aim* in your picture it's A.M., if you don't, it's P.M.

Suppose you take Altace at 11:00 A.M. every day. (Please understand that I'm making these things up arbitrarily in order to teach you the strategy. I'm not a doctor.) Connect *tide* to *old ace*; perhaps many gigantic aces with gray beards are coming in with the tide.

Try this with the medications you take—you'll be surprised at how well it works. You should be able to come up with a Substitute Word or Thought for the name of any medication, but don't labor over it. If the name seems too long or complicated, use the name of the problem that the medicine is supposed to solve. So, if you want to be reminded to take your asthma medication at a certain hour you can associate *as ma*, *ask ma*, or *ass ma* to the hour. Levothyroxine (*leave the rocks in*) is for a thyroid problem; associating thyroid (*thigh right, tire earth*) to the hour serves the purpose just as well.

Just as when you are forming a Substitute Word or Thought for a person's name, that thought or word does not have to sound exactly like the name you want to remember. Always bear in mind that all you need is a *reminder*. I had to take Protonix every morning for a while. In the ridiculous image I created, I was trying to take photos of a gigantic *bee*, but the bee wouldn't let me, it kept *nix*ing the photo. *Photo nix bee* or *bee photo nix* reminded me to take my Protonix pill every morning at nine o'clock. For a while I was taking eye drops every day at 3:00 P.M. and 10:00 P.M. I didn't bother with a Substitute Word for the technical name of the drops, didn't have to. I simply connected "eye drops" to *ma* and *toes*.

Day and Time

If you really feel you need to get more specific, you can make up images that represent both the *day* and the *time of day*. I'll go over that for you and then talk about how to use this strategy, because, as usual, one strategy can solve different, seemingly unrelated memory problems.

The system is really an obvious one, now that you know the basics. You use what I call "compartment" words. Each word will tell you both the day—that is represented by the first consonant—and the hour, which is locked in by the next, the only other, consonant. So, *tide* can only represent Monday (the first day of the week) at one o'clock. *Rock* can only represent Thursday (fourth day) at seven o'clock; *coal* is Sunday at five o'clock. I've already discussed the handling of A.M. and P.M.

What remains is the "handling" of 10:00, 11:00, and 12:00. We already talked about 10:00: use the *s* for zero. *Mouse* represents Wednesday (third day) at 10:00; *cheese* is Saturday (sixth day) at 10:00.

For 11:00 and 12:00, you can make up a word/image that stays within the pattern. For example, the word *rotate* must represent Thursday (fourth day) at 11:00. Make sure you see why this is so. *Mitten* can only represent Wednesday at 12:00—and so on. Here is a list of words you might use.

Monday at 11:00 – doted, toted
12:00 – tighten, titan, deaden
Tuesday at 11:00 – knotted, knitted, noted
12:00 – Indian, antenna
Wednesday at 11:00 – mated, imitate, matted
12:00 – mitten, maiden, mutton

Thursday at 11:00 – rotate, raided, ratted
12:00 – rotten, written
Friday at 11:00 – lighted, loaded
12:00 – Aladdin, laden
Saturday at 11:00 – cheated, jaded
12:00 – shut in, jitney
Sunday at 11:00 – coated, cadet
12:00 – kitten, cotton

Select from my suggestions or make up your own fits-the-pattern word/image. If you use them, they'll be like your Peg Words; you'll know them *because* you use them. There are other ways to handle 11:00 and 12:00, but there's no need for me to take up space teaching them—this one will suffice. Simple idea: get *Aladdin* (rubbing his magic lamp) into your picture and you have your reminder that whatever else is in that picture happens on Friday at 12:00.

Now that you have "compartments" for each day and each time, put the Substitute Word or phrase for each of your medications into the proper compartment.

You're going to have to make choices as to which strategy to use. The *day/time* idea comes in handy when you're taking a *weekly* medication. If you need to take your Actonel once a week, and you decide to do it every Tuesday at 11:00 A.M., form a ridiculous mental picture of *act on L* and *knitted* (or *knotted*). If you want to remember to take your Fosomax every Thursday at 5:00 P.M., associate *fuss oh Max* or *fuss on ax* to *roll*. (Remember what I told you about pronunciation: it needn't be exact.)

Each day, all you need to do is mentally "recite" your words for that particular day. It's Thursday morning, so you think, "roof, rope, rose, rotate, rotten, rod, rain, ram, rower, roll..." Hold it—*roll*. That reminds me that I take my Fosomax at 5:00 P.M. today. (Obviously, you don't take it at 5:00 A.M.) Of course, you'll go over these "Thursday" words a few times that day, so as you get close to 5:00 P.M., you'll be reminded again.

What About the Month?

I know of at least one pill that's taken once a month: Boniva. It's easy to set up a reminder for yourself. Select any word that is *different* from your day/time compartment words and that fits the pattern. It can be any word because, in this case, you won't need that word to remind you of the medicine, you'll need the *medicine to remind you of the word*. So assume you want to take the pill on the nineteenth of every month. Form your silly picture between, say, *tape* (or *tube* or *type*) and your "reminder" word for Boniva, perhaps *bow never, bone ever*, or *bone Eva*). Then, during any month, every time you think of Boniva, you'll be reminded of the *19th*.

On-Time Appointments

I told you that there'd be another use for the strategy I've taught you here. You're probably already aware of it. Since you can now visualize times of any day, you can be reminded of things you have to do at certain *times*. Earlier in the book I talked about Linking your errands and appointments on a daily basis, and that's fine, that may be all you need. It's up to you to apply the strategy that fits into your way of life. But perhaps this will come in handy.

Your dental appointment is for Monday at 9:00 A.M. Associate *tub* to dentist. You can "see" the dentist pulling a tub out of your mouth instead of a tooth, or your dentist is working on you in a large *tub* instead of in his office. At 2:00 P.M., you have to stop at your bank. Your reminder could be a ridiculous mental image of *tin* being deposited at your bank instead of money, or all the bank tellers are large *tin* cans. At 5:00 P.M., you must pick up your car at the garage. Just connect the "compartment" word for day and time (*tail*) to car or garage. And so on.

Understand that if an appointment comes up for later in the week, you can still make the proper association. Assume you were just told that your new prescription eyeglasses will be ready at 2:00 P.M. on Thursday. Your mental image might be *rain*ing eyeglasses.

On Wednesday at 6:00 P.M., you're meeting Mr. Vaikovitch for a drink. You're going to *wake a witch* with a lighted *match*, and you're doing it in a bar. If you don't want to bother with a Substitute Word or Thought for the person's name, you can just as easily visualize having drinks with a bunch of lighted matches.

Okay, it's Sunday evening. Go over all your day/time compartment words for tomorrow, Monday, and you'll know what you have to do tomorrow. You'll come to *tub* and immediately be reminded of your dental appointment and you'll set your clock accordingly. You'll come to *tin* and you're automatically reminded of your bank appointment. You'll come to *tail*, and you'll *know* that you have to pick up your car at five o'clock. If you think of something else that you want to do tomorrow, make your "reminder" association now. When you're brushing your teeth Monday morning, go over the Monday words again—just as a last-minute reminder. It's important to do it before you leave your house so that you're also reminded to take whatever you might need for your various appointments.

Just so that you have it all in one place, here are your compartment words for the week: I'll start each one at 8 o'clock in the morning and go to 1:00 A.M.

Monday: dove (first day, 8:00 A.M.), tub, toes, doted, tighten, tide, tin, tomb, tire, tail, dish, dog…dove, tub, toes, doted, tighten, tide…brings you to 1:00 A.M.—time to go to bed!

Tuesday: knife (second day, 8:00 A.M.), knob, nose, knotted, Indian, net, nun, name, Nero, nail, notch, neck…knife, knob, nose, knotted, Indian, net…

Wednesday: movie (third day, 8:00 A.M.), mop, mouse, mated, mitten, mat, moon, mummy, mower, mule, match, mug…movie, mop, mouse, mated, mitten, mat…

Thursday: roof (fourth day, 8:00 A.M.), rope, rose, rotate, rotten, rod, rain, ram, rower, roll, roach, rock…roof, rope, rose, rotate, rotten, rod…

Friday: leaf (fifth day, 8:00 A.M.), lip, lace, lighted, Aladdin, lot, lion, lame, lure, lily, leech, lake…leaf, lip, lace, lighted, Aladdin, lot…

Saturday: chef (sixth day, 8:00 A.M.), ship, cheese, cheated, shut in, sheet, chain, chum, cherry, jail, choo-choo, chalk…chef, ship, cheese, cheated, shut in, sheet…

Sunday: cave (seventh day, 8:00 A.M.), cap, case, coated, kitten, cot, coin, comb, car, coal, cape, coke…cave, cap, case, coated, kitten, cot…

If an appointment is on a "half hour," you can stick a *half* grapefruit into your picture. That's my standard for "half." For a quarter after an hour, include a quarter (the coin) in your picture. You can use three-quarters of a pie (a slice missing) to remind you of forty-five minutes after an hour. You can get as specific as you like. You can even include a word to remind you of exact minutes. I never bother. If I have to catch a plane at 6:38, I'll use the "grapefruit" idea so that I think of it as 6:30. I'd just as soon give myself a bit of a "cushion" of time, anyway.

This brings me to the end of this chapter, and—it's about time!

SPECIAL MIND-POWER EXERCISE #21

Quite frankly, I've never yet had anyone give me the answer to this one. Yet, it's a fairly easy problem to solve, if you look at it the right way.

The number *four* is unique. In all of "numberdom," there is *no other* number about which you can make this claim.

Your problem, your mind-power exercise, is to see if you can figure out its "uniqueness."

This is not a trick question—it has a legitimate answer.

CHAPTER 22

Speak to Me!

**In lists of "worst fears," death is not number one—
getting up in front of an audience to deliver a speech is!**

Yes, delivering a speech is the number one fear in people's minds. I can help push that fear lower down the list. I'm no psychologist, so I can't talk to you about how to eliminate stage fright in general. I can tell you that, so far as I'm concerned, stage fright is all about forgetting what you want to say. That is certainly so when it comes to "speechifying." It all boils down to *the fear of forgetting what you want to say*! And *that's* an area I *can* talk to you about.

Good speakers do not attempt to memorize their speeches word for word. They understand that verbatim memorizing can get them into trouble. Why worry about one specific word when there are many others that would suffice? We can assume that the person making the speech knows what he is talking about—that's why he was asked to make the speech in the first place! Since he knows what he has to say, he need only memorize the *thoughts* of the speech. And he need only fear omitting a *thought*. (That reminds me of the itinerant preacher who ended up reciting the best parts of his speeches to his horse. In other words, he forgot what he intended to say when in front of the congregation, but remembered it as he was riding away.)

If you *read* your entire speech word for word, you're a bad speaker—because, unless you're a real pro, your audience will know that you're reading. You won't be making proper eye contact with them, for one thing. (Looking up every so often doesn't really fool anyone, and when you look up and then down again,

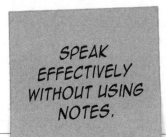

SPEAK
EFFECTIVELY
WITHOUT USING
NOTES.

you may lose your place and have to do a little hem-and-haw dance!) They'll probably think to themselves that you could have mailed them a copy of your speech, to read at their leisure!

Good speakers make reminder notes, which is all right—unless you misplace those notes. Then you're in the position of the poor guy I wrote about in chapter 2 who stammered, "My friends, when I arrived here this evening only God and I knew what I was going to say. Now only God knows!" Mentioning that chapter reminds me to remind you of how ancient orators remembered the thoughts of their speeches, *in sequence*, by using *loci* (places).

Well, it is no longer necessary to associate each *thought* with a different *place*. We're centuries past that. We've made great strides in every area including memory, and now, instead of roaming through a building or home to commit something to memory, all you have to do is form a simple Link!

Key Words Are Key

Okay, you know what you want to say. You've either written out your speech or it's been written and given to you. You want to be reminded of the thoughts of the speech in sequence. (Obviously, remembering them out of sequence would make for a silly speech.)

The *key* here is *key words*. Go over the first thought of your speech, which may be expressed in two, three, or more sentences, even an entire paragraph. Then select one word or phrase, one *image*, that you feel will *bring that entire thought to mind*! If you've ever had to deliver a speech, you know that this is a simple matter. In every thought there *must* be one word or phrase that will bring that entire thought to mind. You can underline that key word, if you like.

When you have selected that word or phrase—the *key word*—do the same with the next thought of the speech. Now you're ready to start forming your Link, exactly as you already know how to do. Continue forming your Link up through the final thought of your speech.

If you wrote your key words, the ones you Linked, on an index card, that card can serve as your notes. But if you've made your Link, why bother with a written list? You don't need it. Just think of the first key word of your Link, which will remind you of the first thought of your speech. Talk about that thought, say it "as it is" as you look at your audience, not at a piece of paper. Then, that first item of your Link will simply remind you of the next thought that you want to talk about.

I'll give you one simple example. What follows is an excerpt from a talk delivered at a PTA meeting. It's "simple" because only four key words are used to recall the entire excerpt. Read it over once and you'll see what I mean.

Ladies and gentlemen, fellow parents:

I'm sure that you're already aware of the problems that exist at this school, including the crowded condition of the classrooms. It's a situation that has existed for some time now.

CROWDED
Some of the classrooms are occupied by twice as many students as they were originally built to handle. Busing students to other schools hasn't relieved the situation because the same number of students is being bused here. Have you taken a good look at some of the seats and desks used by our children? That is, when they're lucky enough to occupy a seat and desk?

FURNITURE
In a recent survey, just about every third seat and every third desk was in extremely poor condition and was scheduled to be replaced. That has still not happened. We've received a few estimates for repairing or replacing all damaged seats and desks, but so far no action has been taken. I don't think I have to tell you about the terrible condition of many of the blackboards in the classrooms.

SALARIES
We have fine teachers here, but I'll be surprised if they stay with us. You know that their salaries are low. They all have to moonlight, and almost all of them are thinking of changing careers or going to different areas where teachers earn higher

salaries. Aside from ourselves, the parents, our teachers are the most important people involved in the upbringing and teaching of our children. At times, they are more important than we are. And yet they each earn less than the person who takes care of your car, your hair, your teeth, your insurance, your clothes, or your plumbing! This situation must be remedied if we value the welfare and well-being of our children.

FIRE
Did your child tell you about the fire-drill fiasco of last week? Were you told that one of the alarms simply didn't sound and that many teachers and children were not aware that a fire drill was in progress? Did you know that one exit door was stuck and couldn't be opened? Many children had to be led to another exit, an exit that was already crowded with students and teachers. Had there really been a fire, you can all imagine the tragedy that might have occurred.

And so on.

If you were the person delivering this speech, the four Linked key words (shown in caps and bold) would have *delivered the speech to you.* You would have formed a Link of those key words, as I've taught you to do. You would make **CROWDED** remind you of **FURNITURE**, perhaps by visualizing a place so *crowded* with *furniture* that you can't squeeze in.

Then you would make **FURNITURE** remind you of **SALARIES**. Perhaps you'd see yourself paying *salaries* (money) to many different pieces of *furniture.*

Next, you could link **SALARIES** to **FIRE**: money burning would surely do it.

If you wanted to go on to talk about the subjects being taught in your school, you might include an image of **SUBJECTS** in your Link. Adding **PLAYGROUND** would remind you to state your opinion about that—and so forth.

A Link formed by a speaker at a convention of dealers, merchants, and store owners might be **PROFIT MARGIN** to **WALK IN** to **GOOD NAME** to **NATIONAL ADVERTISING** to **NEW LINE** to **BREAD AND BUTTER** to **COME BACK.**

Let's say his speech is about the drop in profits over the past couple of years, and what to do about it. He talks about how the **PROFIT MARGIN** has been reduced because of the rise in cost of material, and how to compensate for that.

Then he describes a way to get more people to **WALK IN** to the stores, how to build up the **GOOD NAME** of the company, and ways to combine local advertising with **NATIONAL ADVERTISING**. He talks about his company's **NEW LINE** and how that should help, the importance of making **BREAD AND BUTTER** sales—how to make the customer purchase more than just what he came in for, e.g., holding a two-for-one sale. Finally, he reminds his listeners that the most important thing is to make customers **COME BACK.**

The speaker knows what he wants to say about each thought, each thing covered in the speech. Forming the Link assures that he won't omit an entire thought.

The start of the Link could be a ridiculous picture of his *ma* drinking *gin* and being paid to do so, she's making a "profit" (ma gin/profit; profit margin). His ma *walks in* to many stores; his gigantic name or business card or *good name* is on television or on the cover of a *national* magazine (being nationally advertised); a long line of shiny new magazines (*new line*) are coming off the presses; there's a long, moving line of slices of *bread (buttered)*, and he calls one gigantic slice so that it *comes back* to him.

Once the speaker forms the Link, he is able to approach the podium without notes, without fear, and *with* full confidence.

If he wanted to list the items of the "new line," he'd form what I call an *offshoot* Link. After forming the basic Link, he'd go back to *new line* and start an offshoot Link from that. Let's say the items are Starbright, Holly, Baby Soft, Meteor, and Honeymoon. A shiny new line of *bright stars*, are growing like *holly*, *babies* are growing like *holly* (or you're cradling a gigantic sprig of *holly* as if it were a *baby*), a gigantic *baby* is zipping across the sky like a *meteor*, a bride and groom are zipping back and forth across the sky like a *meteor*—it's their *honeymoon!*

If the new items had style numbers and he wanted to mention them in the speech at the proper time, no problem. Knowing the Phonetic Alphabet takes care of that. Holly is style number 7912, so he'd associate *holly* to *captain*. If there were a letter involved, say, A7912, he'd get "ape" into the picture (the *captain* is an ape!). That's one way to use the "alphabet words."

Word for Word

I know that some of you will think, "Hey, that's fine. But what if I need or want to remember my speech word for word?" Well...you'll just have to work a bit harder, as you would if you weren't applying my techniques. Form the same kind of Link but go over your speech more carefully, more often, more thoroughly. To repeat: my systems are aids to your true memory. When you apply the Link, it forces you to *focus your attention* on the thoughts and *words* of the speech; it forces you to concentrate. The Link enables you to remember the main points; the *ifs, ands,* and *buts* will fall into place automatically.

SPECIAL MIND-POWER EXERCISE #22

Lay out ten markers as shown below. Coins are fine. (Think of the layout as an arrow pointing upward.)

The problem is to move only three of the markers and make the arrow point downward.

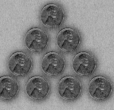

CHAPTER 23

Most Important: Reading/Learning

**How quickly you get through reading material is immaterial.
What's material is how much of the material gets through to you.**

Before we get into the all-important subject of retaining what you read, I want to add one more thing about speaking. The same strategy that I explained in the preceding chapter on speeches can be applied to scripts and lyrics, which usually must be remembered word for word. As I told you, you'll need to go over them more often than you would an "off-the-cuff" speech (which would be true whether or not you were applying my systems). But Linking key words makes it so much easier.

Way back in chapter 2, I quoted from a letter to me from Academy Award–winner Anne Bancroft. That letter, among others, is framed on my office wall. To enlarge on the part I used, the first two paragraphs read: "My most recent play would not have opened had not your systems made it possible for me to memorize an almost impossible-to-memorize script. Not only did it make an impossible task possible but it made what is a usual drudgery part of the creative art.

"I would never have believed that memorizing lines could be as exciting, stimulating, and as much fun as acting itself! You are a Miracle Worker."

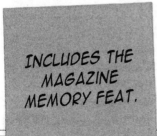

INCLUDES THE
MAGAZINE
MEMORY FEAT.

Part of one of the lines in the script Annie talks about here was, "whether the soldiers cross the bridge."

She kept saying, "*if* the soldiers cross the bridge," which means the same, but the director wouldn't allow it. Annie asked me how she could remember to say "whether." I said, "Tell me, Annie, what's the first thing that comes to mind when I say 'whether'?" She immediately said, "Snow"! She thought "weather" instead of "whether." I said, "Good, visualize soldiers crossing that bridge in a *snowstorm*." She did. Problem solved. When she thought of "soldiers crossing the bridge," she also thought of "weather," and automatically said, "whether the soldiers cross the bridge."

The play was called *John and Abigail.* It was a two-person play in which John and Abigail Adams read from letters they'd sent each other during the Revolutionary War. There were many non sequiturs. At one point, John said, "The cannons are roaring on Beacon Hill," and Abigail's (Annie's) next line was, "The children have the measles." How was Annie to remember that line? John's line didn't give a clue. I told her to visualize the cannons roaring, many tiny cannonballs flying out of the cannon's mouth—and those tiny cannonballs were hitting the faces of the children, causing measle spots or rashes. Again, problem solved; when Annie heard about the "cannons roaring," she immediately knew her next line was about the children having the measles.

Now, onward to the subject of reading.

It's Not How Fast, It's How Well

Many years ago, just for kicks, a strong proponent of "speed reading" challenged one of my students to a reading contest. Each was given the same article to read. The speed-reading "expert" finished much faster than my student (after moving a hand left to right and down each page). But then they were tested. They were asked questions about some of the important information contained in that article. My student scored much higher, *two and a half times* higher. That's what I mean by the quote at the start of this chapter. The fastest way to read is to have to read the material only once!

This chapter follows the chapter on remembering speeches, although remembering what you read is much more important. I don't know how many people reading this book now and (I hope) over many years to come, are "speech makers," but all of them are *readers*. And most of our information and knowledge is acquired through reading—even in our current "Internet world." (After all, you still have to *read* from your screen or printout.)

Reading to Remember

Educator William Lyon Phelps once said, "I divide all readers into two classes, those who read to forget and those who read to remember." I want to ease you gently, but firmly, into the latter "class."

I'm not referring to reading for enjoyment, I'm talking about remembering the *facts* you read that you *want* to remember. (Although my system is a help with pleasure reading, too. An elderly friend of mine was talking about the novel *Gone with the Wind*, and he wanted to mention the author. He stared into space for a couple of moments, then exclaimed, "Darn it; I know it so well, and I've known it for so long—and damned if I can think of her name!" It was a classic "senior moment." I said, "Make this silly picture in your mind: a baseball catcher is wearing a gigantic *shell* instead of his catcher's *mitt* [mitt shell—Mitchell] and a strong wind blows it away; it's gone with the wind. If you think you need to be reminded of Margaret, get a Margarita into the silly picture." Remember, I'm talking about momentarily "losing" bits of information we *know well*. Anyway, he's never again "forgotten" that Margaret Mitchell wrote *Gone with the Wind*, not for any kind of moment, "senior" or otherwise.)

I'm going to use three different articles, each with quite a bit of information, as examples. You may not want to "do" them one immediately after another. Remember, I'm using them only as examples, for teaching purposes, to make sure you understand the strategy. Read this first excerpt:

GREECE
Across the Mediterranean Sea from Egypt is a rocky peninsula with an uneven coast. This is the mainland of Greece.

The first Greeks probably came to the region about 2000 BC. By 1500 BC, they had founded a civilization. They knew how to write and paint, and they built great palaces. But they spent most of their time fighting. About 1100 BC, they were conquered by other Greek tribes who were not so civilized.

If you were interested in this information, you'd probably read it again, this time searching for and forming a Link of the important facts. And by "important," I mean what *you* wanted to remember. For teaching purposes, let's assume you want to remember all of the facts, so let's Link them. Work with me; I'll give you a quick test afterward.

Start your Link with the heading; you can use *Grease*. Headings are important. It depends on what you're reading, of course, but many times just Linking headings and/or bold type will remind you of many important pieces of information. In this case, we'll Link the essential points, starting with the Substitute Word, *grease*. Let's go:

There's lots of grease on a *cross* (across); the cross *meditates* in the middle of the *sea* (Mediterranean Sea) then swims away from a gigantic *pyramid* (Egypt or *gypped*) to a gigantic *rock* on which a gigantic *pen* is writing *unevenly*. Then the pen *coasts* (rocky peninsula, uneven coast), *land*s on a lion's *mane*, which is all *greas*y (mainland of Greece).

You might want to review the above. This part of the Link reminds you that across the Mediterranean Sea from Egypt is a rocky peninsula with an uneven coast. This is the mainland of Greece. Got it? Let's continue.

Many *noses* come out of the lion's mane, one screaming that it was *first* and that it's going to *sue* (noses sue—2000 BC). This will remind you of the first Greeks, who probably came to the region in 2000 BC. If you feel the need, get a Bic pen into your picture to remind you of BC, although that's probably unnecessary since you know that it can't be 2000 *AD*.

A gigantic *towel sees* (1500 BC) the noses and covers them. It's a *civilized towel,* so it starts *writing and painting.* See many people writing and painting on *great palaces* (or people are writing and painting palaces on the gigantic towel). The people doing the writing and painting are continually *fighting* with each other (the people spent most of their time fighting). An *uncivilized tot* and its *sis* (tot sis—1100 BC; although just *tot* would be enough to remind me of the date) conquer all of the people who are fighting.

Go over the Link; you'll probably want to insert some of your own images or change some of mine. Then try to fill in these blanks:

Across the _____ ____ from _____ is a rocky _____ with an _____ coastline. This is the _____ of Greece.

The first Greeks probably came to the region about _____ BC. By _____BC some of them had a _____ (or were _____ _ed); they started ____ing and ____ing, and they built great _____s, but they spent most of their time _____. About ____ BC, they were _____ed by other Greek tribes who were not so _____ed.

If you formed a strong Link originally, you should have breezed through this test. If not, go over the Link again then try this:

Some Greeks had a civilization in ____BC. The Greek Islands are in the _____ Sea. What happened about 1100 BC? (_____ _____ ____). The coastline of Greece is an _____ coastline. The first Greeks arrived in the area about ____BC. The country across the sea from Greece is _____. They wrote and painted, but spent most of their time _____.

Even though I mixed up the questions a bit, you should have had no problem filling in the blanks. That's important for you to know. Once you know the material, even though you have used a Link— which is basically for sequential information—you will know the facts in any order. Here's the next article.

HOW TO MAKE A BAROSCOPE

You will need a quart-size fruit jar and a bottle with a long narrow neck like a soda bottle. First, fill the fruit jar half full of water. Then put a bit of water in the soda bottle and put the bottle quickly upside down into the fruit jar.

Lift the bottle slowly to let a bit of the water out. The bottle should then stand upright in the jar.

When a storm is coming, the air in the bottle will push the water in the bottle's neck down. When the weather is going to be good, the water in the bottle's neck will rise.

Form a Link of the important steps. Start with a picture of a baroscope, if you can. If not, use a Substitute Word or phrase like *bar o' soap* or *barrows cope*. The Link might form as follows: A bar o' soap is washing the *wart (quart)* on a large piece of *fruit* (fruit jar). A large fruit is squeezing into the *neck* of a *soda bottle*. A gigantic soda bottle pours nearly all its liquid into a jar that has half a grapefruit in it. (Half a grapefruit is my standard picture to remind me of "half." Use whatever you like, of course.) Only a little bit of water is left in the soda bottle.

"See" a gigantic soda bottle doing a *quick* dive, landing *upside down* in a gigantic fruit jar. The soda bottle tries to lift itself out but can only lift itself a short distance as some of its water escapes. Then it stands *upright*.

Visualize a *storm* raging over the upside-down soda bottle, which forces the soda bottle to move *down*. Then see the sun come out and the soda bottle moving up to meet it.

I've used the first images that came to my mind. As usual, you may use different ones, which is fine, as long as they remind you of the information. This was pretty easy. If you're with me, let's try something more difficult, involving more information, numbers, etc. First, read it over to get the gist of it.

VENEZUELA

Capital: Caracas
Area: 352,142 square miles
Population: 9,189,280

Venezuela has a long, irregular coastline on the Caribbean Sea. Its neighbors are Guyana, Brazil, and Colombia. It consists of 72 islands. One of the islands, Nueva Esparta, is an important pearl center.

One of Venezuela's rivers is the Orinoco River.

Angel Falls, 3,212 feet high, was discovered in 1937.

Venezuela's chief industries are agriculture, mining, fishing, and raising livestock. It is also one of the world's leading producers of oil.

Its monetary unit is the bolivar; its rate of exchange is (or was at one time) 4.40 per U.S. dollar.

I appeared in front of corporate people in Venezuela for an entire month many years ago. I memorized this information at that time, among many other things. Work along with me, see the mental images. I will test you later.

First, see yourself standing near a body of water, waiting for a whale, asking, "When is the whale here?" That sounds like Venezuela, so a *whale* can be your "heading" picture.

See the whale eating *crackers* (Caracas). *Melon train* might remind you of 352,142. So, see a train that's made of crackers and that's overloaded with melons—it's a melon train. If you think you need something to remind you that *melon train* tells you the "area," see the train covering a lot of area, or get "airy" into your picture. Now, make *melon train* lead you to the population.

A gigantic *bee* (9) swoops down on the melon train to steal the melons. It does and it starts to *divvy up* (189) with its friends (other bees). An argument starts and they fight with *knives* (280). The phrase, *bee divvy up knives* gives you the population. The last thing in your mind is *knives.* See yourself using a knife to cut a long irregular gash down a whale's back (long, irregular coastline). Out of the gash comes a man *carry*ing a gigantic *bean* (Caribbean).

Quick review: *Whale* (Venezuela) leads to *crackers* (Caracas); crackers leads to *melon train* (352,142); melon train leads to *bee divvy up knives* (9,189,280); knife leads to "a long irregular coastline." And…

The gigantic bean flies out of the man's grasp and hits a *guy* who is speaking to *Anna* (Guyana); Anna is holding a gigantic *Brazil* nut (or a large chunk of *brass,* for Brazil); a gigantic Brazil nut is sipping a cup of *Colombian* coffee. (If you can't visualize Colombian coffee, use a Substitute Thought like *column be here.*) The last few images will remind you of Venezuela's neighbors, Guyana, Brazil, and Colombia.

A gigantic *coin* (72 islands) flies out of the cup of coffee. There's a large letter *S* at the *center* of the coin and it's made of *pearl.* You try to part that S from the coin but can never do it. *Never S part* reminds you of Nueva Esparta. The made-of-pearl letter S at the center of the coin reminds you that this city is an important *pearl center.*

With an *oar* you try to *knock* off that S (oar knock—Orinoco River). You can see yourself doing this in a *river*, if you feel that's needed. Millions of oars go over a *waterfall* that's as high as a *mountain* (3,212). As the oars hit bottom, some die and become *angel*s. See whatever brings "angel" to mind, perhaps oars with halos (Angel Falls). An angel is drinking from a gigantic *mug* (37). Those last pictures remind you that Angel Falls is 3,212 feet high and that it was discovered in '37. (If you think you need the 19 for 1937 in the picture, see the angel scooping from a *tub* with the mug.)

Now make "mug" remind you of the chief industries: a large tractor (for agriculture) coming out of the mug; a *miner* (mining; a man wearing a hat with a light on it) is driving it. The miner is *fishing* with one hand and lifting goats, sheep, cows, etc., with the other—to remind you of livestock raising. You should be reminded of agriculture, mining, fishing, livestock raising. The tractor (with all the silliness going on) hits a bump in the road and a gigantic geyser of oil shoots into the air. The oil lands on a *bowler* (to remind of bolivar) who gets so angry he *roars* (4.40), to remind you that the bolivar is 4.40 to the U.S. dollar.

Use your own images if you want to, but go over your Link, then see if you can fill in most of the following blanks.

> *The tallest waterfall in Venezuela is _____ ____, and it is ____ feet high. The four chief industries are _____, _____, _____, and _____. There are ___ islands in Venezuela's territory. Venezuela's estimated population is _____. The monetary unit is the _____, and the rate of exchange is _.__ to the U.S. dollar. One of Venezuela's rivers is the _____ River. _____ is the capital city. Venezuela is one of the world's largest producers of ___. The country has an _____ coastline along the _____ Sea. Venezuela's area is _____ square miles. The island of _____ _____ is an important pearl center. Venezuela's three neighboring countries are _____, _____, and _____.*

If you formed the Link I suggested, or a similar one using your own images, you should have been able to fill in the blanks with no problem—even though I asked the questions out of order. There may have been some facts that you already knew, so you didn't need to include them. If you thought you needed a reminder that the three countries mentioned are "neighboring" countries, you could have included a *neigh*ing horse in the Link. I just want you to realize that you can manipulate it all however you like. And, don't worry about the silly pictures running around in your mind forever. If it's information you intend to utilize, as you use it the silly pictures will fade. They fade in direct relation to the information becoming knowledge! It's important to realize that if you apply the system, you'll be reading more effectively right off the bat, because you're forcing yourself to search for the vital or key thoughts within the material. You're concentrating, you're paying attention, you are *focusing your attention.*

"Seeing" Poetry

Poems are more specific, word-for-word specific. If it's a rhyming poem, the rhyme is a memory aid in itself—but many poems don't rhyme. Read this short poem.

The sun peeks out
with one purple eye.
Without a blink
it searches the world,
then noiselessly sighing
it sleeps again.

Easy. Start with a mental picture of the sun peeking out over the horizon with one gigantic eye (the sun peeks out). For a reminder of "purple," use a Substitute Word or Thought, perhaps a purple grape. Or the eye is being pulled and it pays *per pull*. The gigantic eye doesn't blink at all (without a blink), but it holds a searchlight and searches all over (it searches the world). The searchlight sighs heavily, without a sound (noiselessly sighing) then lies down to sleep again (it sleeps again).

Apply the same strategy to any quote you want to memorize word for word. Here's one from Shakespeare's *As You Like It.*

The whining schoolboy, with his satchel
and shining morning face, creeping like a
snail unwillingly to school.

Perhaps picture a schoolboy whining, or if you like, he's drinking *wine*. See him carrying a satchel (or a *sad shell*), or drinking wine from a satchel. See a *face* on the satchel that shines so brightly that it turns night into *morning*, or there's a snail on the face that shines brightly. See a gigantic snail being dragged unwillingly into a school.

Use your own Substitute Words and images. Try it so that you can see how well it all works. Oh, if you need help remembering whose quote this is, and from which work, you can see the snail *shaking a spear* just *as you like it.* I took a bit of space to teach this concept because it is so important.

The Magazine Memory Feat

Now I'm going off on a bit of a tangent—but only a *bit*.

One of the memory feats I've done for audiences all over the world for—good Lord!—over fifty years, is to memorize an entire issue of a current magazine. The loose pages of the magazine (usually *Time*) are distributed before I'm introduced. Then, at various points during the show, someone calls out a page number and I immediately tell him or her what's on that page, in *detail*. I describe the highlights, photos, names of people in the photos, position on the page of photos and headlines, telephone numbers, license plate numbers, anything significant on that page.

It's one of those feats that always elicits oohs, aahs, and wows. Yes, I present it as a demonstration, but my method for doing it can be applied to any kind of book or other source of information.

The basic idea is as taught in this chapter, with the addition of the Peg Words you learned previously. All I do is associate the word for that page number to the highlight of that page. That's really *it*. If the magazine has more than 100 pages—*Time* usually does—you can make up words for pages 101 and up—*toast, test,* or *dust* (101); *dozen* (102); *dismay* or *toss me* (103); *dozer, dicer,* or *tease her* (104); *tassel* or *diesel* (105), and so forth. After you use these for awhile, the word you decide on for any number is the word that will always come back to you when you think of that number.

So, let's say page 42 is a full-page ad for a Chevrolet. Your association might be of a *chef row*ing (or a chef's hat driving a car) in the pouring *rain*. If a license plate is visible (and I know from experience that if it is, the person is going to wait until I describe the page, and then shout, "What's the license plate number?!"), say B4782, get *brake phone* into your picture. You'll know that that *B* is for the letter *b*—or you can use your alphabet word, *bean*, to make it definite.

Page 78 has a large picture of George Bush at the upper left, so think of a *cave* crammed full of *bushes*. The caption of the article is "What Now?" See yourself trying to get into that cave, but you can't because of all those bushes, and you're saying, "What now?" If there's more stuff on that page that you'd like to remember, Link it to your main ridiculous picture.

There's a photo of a horse on page 2, so start out by seeing many horses boarding the ark (*Noah*) two by two. And so on.

Go over the pages and your associations a few times to lock 'em all in, and you're ready to do the "magazine memory feat." Without making any particular effort, you'll even know that the picture of George Bush on page 78 is at the upper left of the page. That's because each time you think of your Peg Word, the image of that entire page will come to mind. And that's because—let me stress again—in order to apply my systems, you've concentrated on that page as you never could before. I've given you the closest thing there is to a photographic memory. You need only try it to prove it to yourself.

And, as usual—what a wonderful mental exercise it is.

SPECIAL MIND-POWER EXERCISE #23

This is *not* an easy one to work out, but just *trying* to solve it is good mental exercise.

You're lost in a land that's inhabited only by "T" people and "L" people. The T people must always tell the *Truth*; the L people must always *Lie*.

You're traveling to Kumbawa and come to a fork in the road. You have no idea which is the right road for you to take. A man is standing at the fork but there's no way to tell if he's a T or an L person. Here's the problem:

Can you ask this person only *one* question that requires a yes or no answer, and find out which is the correct road to Kumbawa?

Remember, the person may be lying or telling the truth. Give it some thought— that's your mental exercise—before turning to the solution.

CHAPTER 24

Deal Me In

**There is really no such thing as a bad memory.
There are only untrained memories and trained memories.**

Many of those "authorities" who tell you to do crossword puzzles
for mental exercise also suggest that you play cards—and that's
fine. We are a nation of card players. I'm continually asked, by
those who do play, how to remember cards. Of course, there is a
way. You now know that it's easy (certainly eas*ier*) to remember
abstract information when you turn that information from
something abstract into something tangible, something that can
be "seen" in the mind's eye.

The problem here is to turn playing cards into "tangibles." Good
news: it is quite easy to do. Knowing the Phonetic Alphabet, the
ten important sounds, is three-quarters of the battle. The next step
is to simply force each card in the deck to immediately conjure up
an intelligible picture or image in your mind. Since there are fifty-
two cards in a standard deck, you'll need fifty-two "card words." If
you ever want or need to remember cards by number, you can do
that with fifty-two of your Peg Words—1 to 52. You already have
those.

Each card word (though not all of the court cards, as you'll see)
begins with the same letter as its suit. Every club card word
begins with the letter C, every heart card word begins with the
letter H; spades, with an S; and diamonds, with a D. The next and
only consonant sound in each word
tells you the value of the card. That's
all you need. That's all a card is: suit
and value. What a simple strategy!
The first letter tells you the suit, the
next consonant sound tells you the
value.

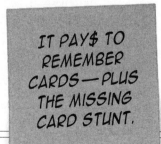

IT PAY$ TO
REMEMBER
CARDS—PLUS
THE MISSING
CARD STUNT.

Look at, think of, the word "cat." Applying the simple strategy I just explained, *cat* can represent only one card in the deck, there are no decisions to make. Do you see which card it represents? It must represent a club card because it starts with a *C*, and it must be a 1—an ace—because the next consonant, the *t*, represents 1 in our Phonetic Alphabet. So *cat* which, of course, you can easily visualize, can represent only that one card, the ace of clubs (AC).

Moving on, *can* begins with a *C* for *c*lubs, and the n sound is 2. *Can* must represent the two of clubs (2C). The word, or picture *ham* can represent only the 3H because it begins with an *H* for *h*earts, and the m sound represents 3. *Sock* represents the 7S, *door* represents the 4D. Since there is no "zero" card, we can use the s sound to represent 10; the word for the 10C is *case*. Be sure you understand these examples before you continue. Once you understand them, we can move on. Here are the words, the pictures I use for all of the "spot" cards, aces to 10s. I'll discuss the "court," or picture cards, afterward.

CLUBS	HEARTS	SPADES	DIAMONDS
AC – cat	AH – hat	AS – suit	AD – date
2C – can	2H – hone	2S – sun	2D – dune
3C – comb	3H – hem	3S – sum	3D – dam
4C – core	4H – hare	4S – sore	4D – door
5C – coal	5H – hail	5S – sail	5D – doll
6C – cash	6H – hash	6S – sash	6D – dash
7C – cock	7H – hog	7S – sock	7D – dock
8C – cuff	8H – hoof	8S – safe	8D – dive
9C – cap	9H – hub	9S – soap	9D – deb
10C – case	10H – hose	10S – sews	10D – dose

For *cap*, be sure to see the visor; you want to differentiate between that and *hat*. If you think that will cause you a problem, use *cup* or *cape* for the 9C. As always, it's your choice. For *cuff*, see a shirt cuff or trouser cuff; for *hone*, I visualize a pair of scissors; for *dam*, I see a waterfall; for *hash*, I see a plate of food; for *core*, an apple core;

for *hoof*, a horseshoe; for *hub*, a wheel (hub of a wheel); for *sum*, a page of numbers; for *sash*, a window; for *dash*, a race or racetrack; for *date*, going on a date, the fruit, or a calendar; for *dune*, a sand dune; for *deb*, a debutante; for *dose*, a spoonful of medicine (or just the spoon). These are suggestions only; whatever comes to your mind for a word is the picture you'll probably always use. As usual, you can change any word you like so long as it fits the system and doesn't conflict with any other word or picture.

You've noticed, I'm sure, that some of the card words are the same as your Peg Words. There's no conflict because the duplications occur only with Peg Words over 52.

Now, we can use the same idea for the picture cards. Since a jack is 11, the word *coated* would fit. *Coated* begins with a C for clubs and the "*ted*" transposes to 11. *Stun* would "work" for the QS (S for spades, tn for 12), *daytime* for the KD, and so on. If you want to make up your own word or phrase (*hit me*—KH) for each picture card, that's fine. I use a different idea, a *rhyming* word that begins with the proper suit letter for six of them.

For the jacks, I simply use the suit word, each of which has meaning and can be visualized: for club I see a club; for heart, a valentine; for spade, a shovel; and for diamond, a large diamond. For the QH I visualize a queen, a woman wearing a crown and flowing robes; for the KC I see a king, a man wearing a crown and knee breeches. (It's important to make sure that your pictures of *king* and *queen* are different enough that you never get confused.)

For the remaining six picture cards, I use a word that starts with the same letter as the suit and rhymes as closely as possible with "queen" or "king." Check them out, go over them only a few times and, I assure you, you'll know them. Check out the following:

JC – club	JH – heart	JS – spade	JD – diamond
QC – cream	QH – queen	QS – steam	QD – dream
KC – king	KH – hinge	KS – sing	KD – drink

For *steam*, I "see" a radiator; for *dream*, I see someone sleeping; for *hinge*, I see whatever I'm connecting to the KH being hinged. The images you choose will automatically "lock in" for you.

It's easy enough to practice. Shuffle a deck of cards, then turn them up one at a time and say the card word (aloud or to yourself). You'll be amazed at how quickly those card words will simply *be there* for you. You won't even have to think of the system, you'll simply know the words/images. When I see the 5H I instantly, automatically, see a large *hail* ball. It's not necessary but, if you like, make up a "practice" deck. Mark the proper card word on the back of each card. You can practice by looking at the word, thinking of the card it represents, and then turning over the card to see if you're correct. Then reverse it and look at the face of the card, think of its word, and so forth. When you can go through the deck both ways, without hesitation, you know your card words.

Place Your Order

You can remember cards in order by applying the Link system exactly as you've learned to do—because now each card is a tangible object. For example, you might want to *see* the pictures of the following 10-card Link:

Horseshoes (*hoof*) are racing, doing the 100-yard *dash*; bottles of *cream* are doing the 100-yard dash; you're cutting a bottle of cream in half with a large pair of scissors (*hone*); a pair of scissors is washing itself with *soap*; you're washing a large sparkling *diamond* with soap (or you break a bar of soap in half and there's a large diamond inside, or you're wearing a bar of soap on your finger instead of a diamond; as usual, there are choices). Continue: a gigantic diamond tips its *cap* to you; you open a *safe* and millions of caps are inside (or you're wearing a safe instead of a cap, or a safe is wearing a large cap); you're giving a safe a *dose* of medicine with a gigantic spoon; you're giving a dose of medicine to a large *sock*, or you're putting on spoons instead of socks, or a gigantic spoon is putting on socks. Select one and *see* the silly picture.

If you really visualize the pictures you select, this Link will enable you to remember the 8H, 6D, QC, 2H, 9S, AD, 9C, 8S, 10D, 7S, in that order, forward and/or backward! All you need are your card words. So, if you want to show off, have someone call off ten (or 15 or 20) cards from a shuffled deck; Link them and then demonstrate your amazing memory. If you *really* want to impress friends or family, you can use the Peg System to remember cards in order, out of order, by number. Let's do ten. Really work with me on these—I'll give you a quick test afterward.

A gigantic *tie* (#1) is *sing*ing (tie to KS, sing).

Noah (2) is wearing a dress (*hem*), or empty dresses are boarding the ark two by two.

Your *ma* (3) is doing a *dive* into water.

A large bottle of *rye* (4) is sitting in the *den*.

A gigantic bill (*cash*) is walking the beat like a cop (*law*—5).

You might want to stop here for a moment and review the first five cards. Then continue.

You're wearing large *heart*s on your feet instead of *shoe*s (6).

A *cow* (7) is hoisting the *sail* on a boat, or a cow *is* the sail on a boat.

*Comb*s are growing on a wall like *ivy* (8), or you're using ivy to comb your hair.

A swarm of *bee*s (9) is attacking a *queen*. (Or a gigantic bee is on a throne, it is the queen. Careful here, you don't want to see just a "queen bee," that's too logical.)

All your *toe*s (10) have large bandages on them—they're *sore*.

Did you really try to see these pictures? If you did, you should know the ten cards in order. Just think "tie, Noah, ma, rye," etc. But you also know them out of order and by number. Amaze yourself by filling in these blanks:

Card #4 is the ___; card #8 is the ___; card #6 is the ___; #1 ___; #10 ___; #3 ___; #5 ___; #9 ___; #7 ___; #2 ___. The 5S is at # ___; the 8D is # ___; the 6C is # ___; 4S # ___; KS # ___; 3C # ___; 3H # ___; QH # ___; JH # ___; 2D # ___.

Obviously, you can "do" fifteen or twenty cards this way. One of the demonstrations I do is to have a whole deck shuffled; then someone calls off all fifty-two cards in order. Then I ask the person I want to impress to call out any number from 1 to 52 and I tell him which card is in that position. Next, I have him call out the name of any card and I tell him which position it is in! You can do this with twenty cards, or with half the deck, or you can remove all the picture cards and do it with the remaining forty.

Great! You'll impress the heck out of people and get some good mental exercise at the same time!

The Missing Card Stunt

But wait. What I want to teach you now is a *strong* demonstration of card memory that's easier than the two already discussed. And it's a concept that you can use when playing cards. I call it the "missing card" stunt, and it uses a "mutilation" strategy.

Dick Cavett hosted one of my television infomercials for a memory-training product. On the show he explained that this was one of his favorite feats and that he uses it often to impress people. The "feat" is this: Your friend removes any five cards from the deck and pockets them. Then he calls off the remaining forty-seven cards at a fairly rapid pace. And—you tell him the names of the five cards in his pocket!

Since you don't use either the Link or Peg system for this, it can be done pretty rapidly (assuming that you know the card words *well*). What you do is to mentally *mutilate* each card word in some way. That's all. So, the 7S is called—see a hole in the *sock*. *Hail* (5H) is called—see a large hail ball melting or falling apart; the 4H is called—visualize a *hare* with only one ear; 4D—you're punching a hole through a *door*, and so on. Just to prove a point, let's try this with one suit, thirteen cards.

If you've tried the preceding Link and Peg examples, you may want to rest your mind a bit before you try this. Lists in sequence or out of order, by number, tend to fade pretty quickly, particularly if you're using them only as a show-off demonstration. If you're using them to retain important information, they fade as you use that information and it becomes knowledge. If you're ready, work with me.

The 6C is called: visualize a large bill (*cash*) being torn in half; the KC: the *king* has been assassinated, he's lying on the floor, bleeding; 2C: see a crushed *can*; 8C: see a torn trouser or shirt *cuff*, AC: picture a *cat* with only three legs or without a tail; 9C: the visor of a *cap* is torn halfway off and dangling; 3C: a *comb* has most of its teeth missing or it's broken in half; QC: a bottle of *cream* is lying on its side as cream spills out of it; 5C: a large lump of *coal* is falling apart, into pieces; 10C: I picture a wooden crate for *case* and see it falling apart, its wooden slats loosening; 7C: a *cock* (rooster) is missing its head.

If you've really "seen" these mutilations, get ready to surprise yourself. You should be able to actually count through a suit of cards—or you *will* be able to do so soon. Cat, can, comb, etc. Try it: Cat (it was missing a leg or tail); can (it was crushed); comb (most of its teeth were missing); core…do you see an apple core with any mutilation? No? Then the 4C must be one of the "missing" (not called) cards. And it is!

Moving on. Coal (it was falling apart); cash (a bill was torn in half); cock (a rooster had lost its head); cuff (a trouser or shirt cuff was badly torn); cap (the visor was torn and dangling); case (a crate was falling apart); club…anything wrong with the club? No? Then the JC is another "missing" card! Finishing up, cream (it's spilling out of its bottle); and, finally, king (he's bleeding on the floor).

Do you see? And do you realize that what the "mutilation" idea is forcing you to do is to *concentrate on each card as you never could possibly do before*? That is the crux of the matter.

When you really know your card words, try this with the entire deck—or cut down on the time it takes by eliminating the picture cards. Have someone remove and pocket any five cards. After the remaining cards have been called off to you, mentally go over your card words suit by suit. It's best always to go through the suits in the same order, so think of the word CHaSeD and it will remind you to go over the suits in this order: clubs, hearts, spades, diamonds.

To impress Bridge players, ask someone to shuffle the deck and then deal out the four Bridge hands. Three of the hands are called off to you—you name every card in the fourth hand.

So, learn your card words and soon you'll be blowing people away with the "missing card" feat—and you'll be training your brain at the same time.

One More Feat

If you want to demonstrate your amazing card-memory ability for a group of people—you'll want at least eight for it to be impressive—try this: Have each person take out two cards from anywhere in the shuffled face-*up* deck. Don't let anyone take pairs, like two nines; that'd be too easy. As each pair is drawn, *connect the two cards*. Example: Someone takes the 3S and 10H; see a large sheet of numbers (*sum*) putting on a pair of *hose*, or there are numbers all over a woman's hose. Another friend takes the JC and 5D. Your quick and silly picture could be of yourself bashing a *doll* with a *club*. Each almost-instant picture "uniting" two cards is a separate and clear one.

When each of the eight people has taken a pair of cards they all hold them so that you can't see the card faces. Now you have choices as to how to demonstrate your fantastic memory. You can ask each person to call out or turn face up one of his cards and you immediately name the other one in his pair. Or you can have someone collect one card from each of the eight people, mix them and hand them to you. Each person then turns his one remaining card face up and you hand each one his or her "partner" card.

You can have someone collect all the cards and mix them thoroughly, and then you lay them out face up in rows, four or five cards in a row. Ask one of the participants to point out the one or two rows that contain his two cards. All you have to do is see which cards in those two rows (or in the one row) are "partner" cards. Those are his two cards—name them. If you see two sets of partner cards, just make one "fishing" statement to find out which is his pair. For example: "You're thinking of one odd-valued card and one even-valued card, right?" Or, "You're thinking of one spot card and one picture card," or "two black cards," etc. The yes or no answer you receive tells you the proper pair.

There are so many ways to present card-memory feats. I could write a book on that alone, but that's not my goal here. Now you know the concept and, more important, you know the card words—so you can devise your own presentations. Using ten or twelve people for the one I've just suggested is much more impressive, of course.

Mutilate and Conquer

Moving in a slightly more practical direction, you can apply what you now know to card games—only for fun, of course. When playing Gin Rummy, for example, it's valuable to know which cards have been played or discarded so that you know if it's safe for you to discard a particular card. As you play, mentally "mutilate" each card that's being discarded, just as I've taught you to do. Then, when it's your turn to discard one of your cards, you don't have to mentally go over all of your card words. That'd take too long.

You need to think of only three or four cards. Assume you want to discard the 6C. Is it safe to do so? Think of your card words for the 5C and the 7C. If they haven't been mutilated, be careful about discarding the 6C—your opponent may be holding the 5C and 7C, just waiting for that 6C to fill a club "run." If the 5C and 7C *have* been mutilated, check the other sixes. If two of them have been mutilated, your opponent doesn't need the 6C to fill a six "lay" and you know that it's safe to discard it.

Also in Gin Rummy, it's valuable to remember which of your discards your opponent has taken. So, whenever he takes one, associate the card word to his, say, nose, or whatever silly picture you think of. Anytime you need to know which cards he took from the discard pile, you'll know them! Doing this makes you *originally aware* of each card he takes, and you can do this during each hand of play without getting confused. Try it, see for yourself.

Apply the idea to Bridge in a way that benefits your particular mode of play. You can mutilate only the trump cards that have been played, or *all* the cards that have been played. It's up to you.

You may be wondering how you can repeat the "missing card" demonstration immediately without getting confused. Well, you shouldn't repeat it immediately unless you change it a bit. Instead of mutilation, use *fire* the next time—that is, "see" each card word *burning*. I mention this here because when playing Gin Rummy or Bridge, you'll be applying the strategy for each hand of play. Using mutilation one hand after another can be confusing. So, use fire; it's a form of mutilation, but different enough so as not to confuse the issue. For the next hand, use *water:* see each card-word image under water, drowning. Then you can use a *knife*: see each image being cut. After that, you can associate each card word to yourself, and so on. After that, you'll be ready to start the cycle all over again.

When I play Blackjack I remember all the high cards, the 8, 9, and 10 counts, which have been played, so that I have a good idea how many *low* counts are still in the dealer's shoe. It's all by average, of course, because they never deal through the entire shoe, which contains anywhere up to six full decks. Anyway, I play and bet using my system, and *win*. There are a few casinos that won't deal Blackjack to me! "C'mon, Mr. Lorayne, let me buy you a drink," that sort of thing. It's all silliness, of course, because after I win at Blackjack, and it's *work*, a grind, I go to the crap table for fun—and lose it all back, plus! (Memory doesn't help me at the crap table, except to remember all the odds. I know them but I pay no attention to them because I'm at the crap table for *fun*.)

Please bear in mind that no matter how well you can remember cards, if you don't understand a particular game thoroughly, it won't help you much. I win at Blackjack because I played the game on the mean streets, right on the sidewalks of the Lower East Side of Manhattan, starting when I was perhaps seven years old. (It was called Twenty-One.) So, I know the game inside out, I know the odds, I know when to hit, stay, split, double down. If you don't really know the game you're playing, be careful. I take no responsibility for your losses! (But feel free to send me a percentage of your winnings!)

SPECIAL MIND-POWER EXERCISE #24

8	11	14	1
13	2	7	12
3	16	9	6
10	5	4	15

This is a magic square for the number 34. All the horizontal rows and all the vertical columns total 34, and so do the two diagonals. But this square goes a bit further than most. The four corners (8, 1, 10, 15) total 34; the four numbers in the upper-left quadrant (8, 11, 13, 2) total 34, as do the upper-right, lower-left, and lower-right quadrants; so do the four numbers in the center quadrant. There are more patterns, but these are enough.

Can you figure out how this magic square was put together, in a way that'd enable you to form just such a square for any number over 34? It's much easier than you might think.

CHAPTER 25

Spelling Bee

"Red Hot You Two-Headed Monster"

My dyslexia manifests itself in strange ways. I won't take your time discussing them except for this one, because it's apropos.

Ever since I was a small boy I haven't, for the life of me, been able to spell the word *rhythm*. I'm a darn good speller otherwise. I solved the problem by making up and thinking of the phrase at the top of this page. I visualize a two-headed monster playing red-hot rhythm. Now, whenever I have to write or type that word, as I just did, I say that phrase to myself so I will spell the word properly. Well, that's fine, it works for me for that one word. But I don't suggest doing that with more than one word, because there are better ways.

Let's face it: as we get older, we may not be that concerned with spelling every word correctly. That's not really the point. My main point is that the concept I'll discuss here is an excellent mental exercise and you may enjoy sharing it with school-age relatives or friends. Or…you may just want to improve your spelling ability—no matter what your age.

I touched on some spelling ideas back in chapter 5, where I mentioned "Never be*LIE*ve a *LIE.*" That phrase helped me spell "believe" correctly when I was a young boy. I've expanded upon that idea a great deal over the years. In that chapter I also taught you how to keep track of the differences between Audrey and Aubrey, Francis and Frances, desert and dessert, stationery and stationary. You might want to go back and refresh your memory.

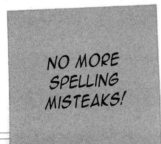

NO MORE
SPELLING
MISTEAKS!

Connecting *believe* and *lie* in my mind was an amazing and immediate help. We hadn't learned the "*i* before *e* except after *c*" rule yet. And there are exceptions to that rule: counterfeit, protein, sheik, caffeine, codeine. If you want to remember the more common exceptions think of these sentences: "A *weird* person *seizes neither leisure* nor pleasure" and "The counter*feit sheik* thought that caff*ei*ne and cod*ei*ne gave him prot*ei*n."

The same idea that enables you to remember the difference between Franc*I*s (h*I*s) and Franc*e*s (h*E*r or sh*E*) can be used for princi*ple* and princi*pal*. I'm amazed at how often I see these words used incorrectly, even in large public advertisements. It's so easy to know the difference. The princi*PAL* is your *PAL*; a princip*LE* is a ru*LE*. Think of these now, and forever hold your peace (not "piece," as in *PIE*ce of *PIE*. If the war will c*EA*se, we'll be at p*EA*ce).

Let's look at *capitol* versus *capital,* another pair that is commonly misused. The spelling with the *O* is used *O*nly when it refers to the building in Washington, D.C., or any capit*Ol* d*O*me. In all other instances, it is spelled with an *A*, as in capit*A*l of a state, or capit*A*l/c*A*sh.

Nav*E*l—b*E*lly button; nav*A*l—n*A*vy (or w*A*ter).

Most spelling errors are habitual. We call that "persistence of error." Remembering the above "connections," and those that follow, will break those bad habits.

Another spelling aid I learned as a boy is "*ALL* lines are par*ALL*el." I've never misspelled that word since. (A *MISS* never *MISS*pells reminds me of the double *s*.) There were others I learned, but mostly I made up my own over the years, to help myself and to teach to others—like you. These are all geared toward spelling "trouble spots." Try to really see the "action" or premise of each in your mind for just a moment.

Don't *EAT* l*EAT*her.

It was a co*LOSS*al *LOSS*.

You *ERR* when you int*ERR*upt.

It is ne*CESS*ary to clean your *CESS*pool.

EIGHT pounds is a w*EIGHT*.

A bar*GAIN* is a *GAIN*.

Your *SECRET*ary has a *SECRET*.

BR, it's cold in fe*BR*uary.

A *BALL*oon is round like a *BALL*.

To *AGE* is no tr*AGE*dy.

An ar*GUM*ent over *GUM*.

A large digit *NINE* wears a dress—it's femi*NINE*.

IRON is part of the env*IRON*ment.

The *CHIEF* causes mis*CHIEF*.

You must show *COURT*esy in *COURT*.

They were *WED* on *WED*nesday.

It's a *FEAT* to balance a *FEAT*her.

It was the *END* of my fri*END*.

There's a *BULLET* on the *BULLET*in board.

You *EA*t a st*EA*k.

A *GUAR*d *GUAR*antees safety.

See if you can devise similar memory aids for these:

Kinderg*art*en, deter*mine*, w*itch*, v*ill*ain, *labor*atory, *bus*iness, per*man*ent, cata*log*, *arc*tic, *ill*ustrate, *pea*sant, capa*city*, fr*eight*, *hand*kerchief, Lo*ray*ne.

A Few More Spelling Aids

There are other aids you can apply. I remember a boy asking for my help because he always spelled it "mo*t*ercycle." I told him to think of himself as the *t* on the motorcycle with the two OOs on either side of him being the two wheels. Look at the word and you'll see what I mean. It solved the problem. As you know, I don't care how silly or ridiculous you get with your pictures. Coming up with them is an imagination, creativity, mind exercise, and you're focusing your attention on the troublesome word at the same time.

To remember something new (or seemingly difficult to remember), associate it to something you *already* know/remember. That's the rule I've been applying all along, and it works for spelling, too. I knew how to spell "lie" when I was a boy; "believe" was the new, troublesome word.

When I wanted to remember that "occasion" is spelled with two *c*'s, I thought, "On oc*ca*sion I have an ac*ci*dent." I knew how to spell "accident," so connecting that to the troublesome "occasion" was enough of an aid.

Think of "all right" as being the opposite of "all wrong" and you'll never again spell it "alright," which is all wrong!

Do you keep spelling it "expence" instead of the correct way, "expense"? Think of the word spelled with a dollar sign at the trouble spot, "expen$e," and you'll be reminded that an *s* goes there.

The alphabet words can also be used as a spelling aid. To remind you that it's "insur*a*nce" not "insur*e*nce," picture an *ape* selling insur*a*nce. See an *eel* having a long exist*e*nce, two *hams* shooting am*m*unition, an *ape* being sep*a*rated, an *eel* performing surg*e*ry, an *ape* getting an allow*a*nce.

Now, you're aware of some of the strategies that it *takes* to avoid spelling mis*takes*!

CHAPTER 26

Bible Study

"To know wisdom and instruction; to perceive the words of understanding."
—Book of Proverbs

Through the years, many of my students have told me how thrilled they are when they realize they can remember Bible facts as they never could before, by applying my trained-memory strategies and techniques. Some have even written books about it—one writing as if *he* devised the ideas! (He even declared that the Lord taught him how to do it, as he used my thoughts and teachings *word for word*. I won't bother to respond to that, except to say, Talk about taking the Lord's name in vain!)

That, of course, is neither here nor there. The fact is, my techniques can be applied to *any* memory problem. Personally, I'm not a student of the Bible, so I can't go deeply into the subject. What I can do is touch on the answers I've given to some questions I've been asked over the years.

A Bible scholar once asked me how to go about remembering the Twelve Minor Prophets. All you need is the ability to form Substitute Words or Thoughts and knowledge of the Link system of memory. Here are the twelve prophets and my first thoughts for Substitute Words.

Hosea – hose, eh; whoa, say yeah
Joel – show L
Amos – aim us; A moss
Obadiah – oh, bad eye; O bad dyer
Jonah – whale; Joan, ah
Micah – my car; mike her
Nahum – nay hum; neigh hum
Habbakuk – have a cook
Zephaniah – savin' eye; seven eye, ah

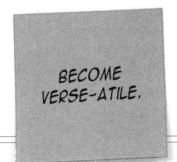

BECOME
VERSE-ATILE.

Haggai – hay gay; hag A
Zechariah – sack awry; sack car eye
Malachi – ma lock key

My assumption is that if you want to remember these twelve Minor Prophets, you must basically know them already; what you need are *reminders*. So Linking *Hose eh* (Hosea) to *show L* (Joel) to *aim us* (Amos) to *oh, bad eye* (Obadiah) to *whale* (Jonah), and on to *ma lock key* (Malachi) will lock them in for you. It sure did for the person who asked me about it. You can, of course, make up your own Substitute Words or Thoughts.

Bible Books

I've also been asked, many times, how I'd go about remembering books of the New Testament. You should know the answer to that by now, too. You can Link the Substitute Word or Thought for each book, or you can use the Peg System to remember them in and out of order, by number. Look:

Book 1: Matthew. Visualize a *ewe* (or letter *u*) doing *math* (*math ewe*; or *mat you*) on a gigantic *tie* (1).

Book 2: Mark. You're *mark*ing up an old man with a long white beard (*Noah*—2), or marking up the ark.

Book 3: Luke. *Look* (Luke) at *ma* (3). Make it silly, you don't want a logical, mundane picture. You can also visualize your ma being *luke* warm.

Book 4: John. Connect a *john* (bathroom; or *yawn*) with a bottle of *rye* (4) whiskey or a loaf of rye bread.

Book 5: Acts. Policemen (*law*—5) are onstage doing their *acts*. *Axe* would also remind you of Acts.

Book 6: Romans. Mark Antony or Caesar, or any Roman is holding a gigantic *shoe* (6). Or a *man* is rowing a gigantic shoe instead of a *row*boat (*row man*). Or, a gigantic shoe is *roamin'* the streets.

Book 7: I Corinthians. *Gorin' the ants* or *core in the ants*. Associate either to *cow* (7). I'd get *won* into the silly picture to remind that it's *one* Corinthians.

Book 8: II Corinthians. Associate *ivy* (8) to one of the above, and get *toot* or *tool* (or whatever you want to remind you of "two") into the picture to remind you that this is *two* Corinthians.

Book 9: Galatians. *Gal ate shins* to *bee* (9). You may have thought of *gala shins* or *gal A chins*.

Book 10: Ephesians. *F feeds E ins* or just *F feeds* should do it for you. *A fee Z Ns, A fee see ants* would also make good reminders. If you don't think you can visualize the letters *f* and *e* use your alphabet words, *half* and *eel*.

If you're really trying to learn these, go over them once or twice to review and they'll become knowledge soon enough.

You can continue learning the Books by number; just make up Substitute Words for Book 11: Philippians (*full lip eons* or *fill lip peons*) to Book 27: Revelations.

If you want to remember the Books of the Old Testament, do the same. You can Link Genesis (*gem is sis* or *Jennie sis*) to Exodus (an exodus, or *exit us*) to Leviticus (*leave it, it cuts, Lefty cuts*) to Numbers (just see lots of *numbers* or, if you prefer, *numb bears*) to Deuteronomy (*due to run on me*) and so on. Connect them to your Peg Words if you want to remember them by number, in and out of order.

Bible Verses

I've always known the 23rd Psalm (The Lord is my shepherd, I shall not want...); I imagine most people do. But do you know the 1st Psalm, or the 2nd or 3rd, or the 24th, 40th, 71st, etc? I don't think I need to go into too much detail here. You already know what to do if, for whatever reason, you'd like to memorize the Psalms by number. (I could have included this in the "One-Upmanship" chapter.)

Just connect your Peg Word for the Psalm's number to the main thought of the Psalm. Again, the assumption is that if you're at all familiar with them, the main thought (or what *you* select as the main thought) will bring the bulk of the Psalm to mind. The following are from the King James Version of the Bible.

For the first Psalm, associate *tie* to "Do not follow the counsel of the wicked…" (or "the ungodly"). That would be the main or basic thought for me. You could visualize a gigantic *tie* saying "No, no" to the "Wicked witch," or whatever you want to include that would mean "wicked" to you. And, if you want to, you can Link other thoughts to this initial silly picture. For example, whatever you select as your mental image of "the Lord and his law" to remind you of "The law of the Lord." Then include a "tree planted by the rivers of water," and so forth.

Psalm 2: Associate *Noah* to "heathens raging."

Psalm 3: Your *ma* has many foes and adversaries against her.

Psalm 8: Much *ivy* is coming "Out of the mouths of babes" (and sucklings).

Psalm 10: *Toes* are standing far off. ("Why standeth thou afar off, Oh Lord?")

Psalm 22: A *nun* is walking away from you, forsaking you. ("My God, why hast thou forsaken me?")

Psalm 27: Visualize a bright light emanating from your (or someone's) *neck*, and it saves your life. ("The Lord is my light and my salvation.")

Psalm 40: A gigantic *rose* is waiting patiently. ("I waited patiently for the Lord.")

Psalm 66: A *choo-choo* train is making a joyful noise. ("Make a joyful noise unto God…")

Psalm 86: A gigantic *fish* is bowing down so that its ear is near you. ("Bow down thine ear, O Lord.")

Psalm 97: You open a gigantic *book* and clouds and darkness fly out of it and overwhelm you. ("Clouds and darkness are round about Him.")

Psalm 121: (I use *tent* as the Peg Word for 121.) Visualize many eyes lifting out of a tent and moving up toward a hilltop. ("I will lift up mine eyes unto the hills.")

Psalm 149: (*Trip* is my Peg Word for 149.) You're taking a trip in order to "sing unto the Lord a new song."

Now that you have the idea, you can apply it to any verse in any version of the Bible.

Godspeed!

SPECIAL MIND-POWER EXERCISE #26

You have coins totaling $1.19 in your pocket. Yet, you can't make change for a dollar, a half dollar, a quarter, a dime, or a nickel!

Your mind exercise is to figure out which coins you have in your pocket. Remember—they total $1.19 but you can't use them to make change for anything.

CHAPTER 27

The 400-Digit Memory Feat

"The memory is always present, ready and anxious to help, if only we would ask it to do so more often." —Roger Broile

	1	2	3	4	5	6	7	8	9	10
A	9491	0261	4850	8210	1427	0214	5390	0141	7450	7590
B	2195	6140	5827	1214	4270	9401	2071	5014	1395	8150
C	8520	7461	9511	7157	9420	4532	7775	1404	7841	7410
D	2116	5120	9470	2154	9750	7471	7220	1941	0191	3102
E	4595	5891	3944	3017	0594	9414	6720	8227	1752	7480
F	0137	5814	9950	9427	1285	2754	2145	1540	8927	9521
G	9015	3145	8195	8540	9514	7040	7312	1211	9227	1270
H	9210	4014	0216	4910	3212	7421	1484	2469	0791	2520
I	4175	1842	3058	7462	9285	0746	6245	7527	0743	3510
J	4952	9434	0941	7212	9402	7213	5810	1204	6920	3062

How would you like to hand a card as above to someone you want to impress, have him call off any letter/number combination— and be able immediately to tell him the four-digit number at that juncture?! Well, you can, and it shouldn't take you more than a couple of hours to learn how. Then you'll know it forever and everyone will think you're a genius!

YOU'VE NEVER REMEMBERED NUMBERS LIKE THIS BEFORE.

What I've done is to make up a

word *that fits a pattern* for every letter/number combination. And a simple pattern it is. The word must start with the vital letter, and the next, the only other consonant sound is the Phonetic Alphabet sound for that number. Here's what I mean: *Ate* is the word for A1. Think of that for a moment or two, and from now on, when you hear A1, *ate* must come to mind. A2 is *awn*, A3 is *aim*, B4 is *bar*, C8 is *cave*, D9 is *dope*, E4 is *err*, F10 is *fuse*, G8 is *gave*, H1 is *hat*, I6 is *itch*, J4 is *jar*. Make sure you understand the pattern.

But how do these "pattern" words help? When I formed the square, I generally used the first word that the "pattern" word easily brought to mind that contained exactly four consonant sounds. For *ate* (A1) I came up with *burped*. I thought, "I ate and then I burped." And *burped* transcribes to 9491 in our Phonetic Alphabet! An *awn* (A2) is a *sunshade:* 0261. *Bar* (B4) made me think of *(bar)tender:* 1214. For some, I couldn't use my first thought because it conflicted with another four-digit number, so I came up with something else.

These are the words I came up with many years ago. I'd think of much better ones now, but the originals are so ingrained, it'd be silly for me to change them. All of my original words are listed below. Look them over and then I'll talk about them some more.

A1: ate – burped	B1: bat – and ball	C1: cat – felines
A2: awn – sunshade	B2: bean – shooters	C2: can – crushed
A3: aim – rifles	B3: bum – loafing	C3: comb – bald head
A4: air – vents	B4: bar – tender	C4: car – Cadillac
A5: ale – drink	B5: bell – rings	C5: coal – burns
A6: ash – cinder	B6: badge – breast	C6: cash – real money
A7: ache – limps	B7: bug – insect	C7: coke – Coca-Cola
A8: ave – street	B8: buff – luster	C8: cuff – trouser
A9: ape – growls	B9: baby – dimple	C9: cap – covered
A10: ace – clubs	B10: bass – fiddles	C10: case – crates

D1:   dot – and dash
D2:   din – loud noise
D3:   dam – breaks
D4:   deer – antler
D5:   dill – pickles
D6:   dish – cracked
D7:   dog – canines
D8:   dove – white bird
D9:   dope – stupid
D10: dose – medicine

E1:   eddy – whirlpool
E2:   en – alphabet
E3:   em – emperor
E4:   err – mistake
E5:   eel – slippery
E6:   edge – border
E7:   egg – chickens
E8:   eve – evening
E9:   ebb – decline
E10: ess – curves

F1:   fat – stomach
F2:   fun – laughter
F3:   foam – bubbles
F4:   fur – bearing
F5:   foil – tinfoil
F6:   fish – angler
F7:   fake – not real
F8:   five – dollars
F9:   fib – fibbing
F10: fuse – blend

G1:   gat – pistol
G2:   gown – material
G3:   game – football
G4:   grow – flowers
G5:   gall – bladder
G6:   gush – geysers
G7:   gag – comedian
G8:   gave – donated
G9:   gap – opening
G10: gas – tanks

H1:   hat – bands
H2:   hen – rooster
H3:   ham – sandwich
H4:   hare – rabbits
H5:   hill – mountain
H6:   hash – corned
H7:   hack – driver
H8:   have – ownership
H9:   hop – skipped
H10: hose – nylons

I1:   it – article
I2:   inn – tavern
I3:   I'm – myself
I4:   Ira – Gershwin
I5:   ill – painful
I6:   itch – scratch
I7:   Ike – general
I8:   ivy – cling
I9:   (y)ipe – scream
I10: ice – melts

J1:   jet – airplane
J2:   John – Barrymore
J3:   jam – spread
J4:   jar – contain
J5:   jail – prison
J6:   judge – condemn
J7:   jack – lifts
J8:   jive – dancer
J9:   Jap. – Japanese
J10: jazz – musician

Go over these a few times, concentrating as you do, and you'll know them in a short while. Here, the *logical* extension is what makes it work, makes it easy. There is no word that begins with an *i* that has only the *b* or *p* sound after it, so I improvised with *(y)ipe* for I9; it works fine. You can change words, of course. For *john*, you could use *toilets* (1510) or *bathroom* (9143). Instead of *Ike* you could use *icky*; instead of *Ira*, you could use *ire*; instead of *en*, you can use *enter*, and so on. Of course, if you do make any changes, you have to make the new "pattern" word remind you, logically, of another word or phrase that transcribes to a four-digit number that doesn't duplicate any other four-digit number.

If your friend asks for a number backward, not a problem. If he calls G5, you think "gall," which leads you to *bladder*. Just visualize 9514, and give him the digits backward. If someone asks for all the D numbers, all you have to do is think D1, then D2, D3, all the way to D10.

This is a feat of memory that simply can't be done without the memory system. You'll have people going over the "graph" looking for a mathematical "secret." They'll never find one, of course, because there is none—it is *memory,* pure and simple. It's just another way you can show off your "ageless memory" for friends and family and exercise your mind at the same time.

SPECIAL MIND-POWER EXERCISE #27

On the left side of a balancing scale are three books. On the right side is one book and one half-pound weight. The scale is perfectly balanced.

The books each weigh exactly the same amount.

The problem: What's the procedure for figuring out how much each book weighs? And how much *does* each book weigh?

CHAPTER 28

Instant, Alternate, Peg Lists

Do you know your ABCs?

I want to be sure you understand that you can use your basic Peg Words over and over again. As I've mentioned before, they work like a child's "magic slate": when you lift the top plastic sheet you have a "clean slate" on which to write all over again. And, if you use the same Peg Words for two different number lists, your mind will know the difference.

But, if and when you like, you can use *different* Peg Word lists. I'll teach you some of them here for the sake of thoroughness (though I'm not going to teach you all of them).

In an early chapter, I mentioned that the ancients used bits of knowledge, such as the signs of the zodiac, for "pegs," just as actors and vaudeville performers used elements of the theater: the orchestra pit, the balcony, the loges, the audience, the exit signs, the chandelier, and so on.

Here's a short Peg Word list I teach to children, who learn it in minutes. It's based on "The Children's Marching Song" that starts out "This old man, he played one, he played knick-knack on a gun…This old man, he played two, he played knick-knack on my shoe," etc. The Peg Words rhyme with the numbers, that's all there is to it. (I didn't want to use "gun" when teaching the list to children, so I've changed it to "run.") Here's the list:

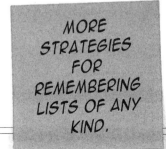

MORE STRATEGIES FOR REMEMBERING LISTS OF ANY KIND.

1. Run	5. Dive	8. Gate
2. Glue	6. Sticks	9. Dine
3. Tree	7. Heaven	10. Hen
4. Pour		

Now all you have to do is "see" the item that you want to remember as #1 *running*. (I've changed a few others from what was in the song to words that are easier to visualize.)

For *heaven*, picture the sky. You can use *line* for 9, if you'd rather. Go over these once or twice and you've got 'em. You might even "have 'em" now, without going over them! That's why I refer to this as an *instant* Peg list.

Assume you want to quickly memorize the following ten items: appointments, errands, thoughts of a speech, main thoughts of an article you're reading, whatever.

#4 (pour) is a *wristwatch*. See watches *pour*ing out of something, or something is pouring out of your wristwatch.

#8 (gate) is *ashtray*. See a large ashtray being a swinging *gate*, see ashes and cigarette butts falling out of it.

#1 (run) is *lamp*. Lamps are *run*ning.

#10 (hen) is *basketball*. See *hen*s playing basketball, or you're dribbling, shooting, a hen instead of a basketball.

#5 (dive) is *mattress*. Imagine a mattress *div*ing into water, or you're diving into (onto) a gigantic mattress.

#9 (dine) is *cell phone*. Visualize yourself *din*ing on cell phones (they're ringing as you dine), or a gigantic cell phone is dining.

#3 (tree) is *book*. See books growing on a *tree* instead of leaves, or you're reading a tree instead of a book.

#7 (heaven) is *car*. Cars are driving all over the sky (*heaven*).

#2 (glue) is *playing cards*. You're dealing cards but they are all *glue*d together, or see playing cards glued all over you.

#6 (sticks) is *toothbrush*. You're brushing your teeth with a bunch of *sticks* instead of a toothbrush. Visualize the sticks causing your gums to bleed.

You should have "done" these quickly, just as quickly as you'll fill in these blanks.

#1 is _____	#6 is _____
#2 is _____	#7 is _____
#3 is _____	#8 is _____
#4 is _____	#9 is _____
#5 is _____	#10 is _____

And, of course, you know them forward, backward, by number, in and out of order, inside out and every which way. It's a short Peg list for emergencies. You can take it to twelve, if you like, using *leaven*ed bread (matzo) for eleven, *shelf* for twelve. I wouldn't go any higher than that.

You may be using *hen* as your "alphabet word" for *n* but that will *not* confuse you. Take my word for it. The mind is a fantastic machine, particularly if you keep it "oiled," as this book is teaching you to do. It will keep your Peg lists *separated*. You'll see that this is so when you actually *use* the ideas. Your mind is the best computer of all!

Alphabet Pegs

I also devised the "alphabet Peg Word list." It's based on *adjectives*. What the adjectives do is force you to instantly know the numerical position of any letter of the alphabet. Once you know that, your alphabet words can be used as an emergency Peg list. In other words, if you associate a *bracelet* to, say, *eye* (for the letter *i*) and if you really *know* that *i* is the ninth letter of the alphabet, then you'll know that *bracelet* is number 9 and number 9 is *bracelet*.

You already know the alphabet words. Here's how to use the adjectives:

Awful tie	**D**elicious rye
Brave Noah	**E**xcellent law
Cute ma	**F**inicky cow

And so on. Make up your own adjectives because the ones you make up yourself will work better for you. You might use *j*agged toes, *k*ind tot, *q*uiet dog, *v*ivacious nun, *x*-rayed Nero, *z*igzag notch. Each (logical, in this case) phrase tells you two things: the letter (the first letter of the adjective) and its *position* (the second [Peg] word of the phrase).

Review your phrases a couple of times and before you know it, when you think *p* you'll also think "plastic *dish*," and you'll instantly know that *p* is the sixteenth letter. So whatever you've associated to your alphabet word for *p* (*pea*) is sixteenth on your list. Interesting, isn't it? You've known and recited the alphabet all your life but you never really knew that *m* is the thirteenth letter (*m*arble *tomb*).

SPECIAL MIND-POWER EXERCISE #28

This will take some thinking (and mental exercise) on your part.

Think of a common English six-letter word from which you can remove one letter at a time, leaving another common English word each time.

That is, remove one letter to leave a five-letter word, remove another letter and leave a common four-letter word, and so on, until you can't remove any more letters.

The letters always remain in the same order.

If you don't want a hint or two, don't look below.

You end with a one-letter word. It's worth a drink if you find the answer in a short time.

CHAPTER 29

Memory Potpourri

"A great and beautiful invention is the art of memory,
always useful both for learning and for life." —Dialexeis, ca. 400 BC

Calories

Are you watching your calorie intake? So many of us are. If you want to remember the caloric content of anything, just apply my system. It's easy.

One fried egg contains 100 calories. Associate egg to *disease* (or *dazes*) and you'll always remember it.

One serving of Cheerios has 110 calories. *Totes* to Cheerios. You might visualize someone *cheer*ing as he *totes* heavy packages. One ounce of instant oatmeal has 105 calories. A large oat (or goat) is driving a *diesel* truck, or wearing a *tassel*.

One Lenders bagel has 250 calories. *Nails* through a gigantic bagel. Associate *bone* to mayonnaise (*mayor*, or *Mayo* Clinic) and you'll know that a tablespoon of the stuff contains 92 calories.

A glass of generic red wine has 75 calories (associate to *coal*); a glass of white wine, 70 calories (associate to *case*); and a glass of Merlot contains 83 calories (associate *mare low* to *foam*). Muscatel has 140 calories (*mouse cat tell* to *tires*, or *doors*). A small glass of champagne is only 80 calories (champagne does *fizz*). An eight-ounce glass of beer has 175 calories (associate beer to *tickle*, *tackle*, or *toggle*). A six-fluid-ounce serving of cola has 80 calories, while an eight-ounce serving has 105: *fuzz* and *tussle*.

REMEMBER CALORIES, WHERE YOU PARKED YOUR CAR, DIRECTIONS, TRIVIA, DATES, AND MORE.

A Hershey bar contains 240 calories (*hearse E* to *no rose, Nero's* or *nears*).

A bacon cheeseburger (yum!) has 400 calories (associate it to *roses, raises*, or *rises*). A medium-size frankfurter has 300 calories (connect hot dog to *muses* or *amazes*). A Whopper with mayo has 670 calories—you can associate it to *chokes* (!). Without mayo, the Whopper is 525 calories (*Lionel* or *lonely*). A Big Mac, 580 calories: *loves, loaves,* or *leaves* to *big Mack.*

Quick Think

In an earlier book I talked about a quick way to remember a five- or six-digit number that you need to keep in mind for only seconds; for example, as you move from computer to paper to write it down. Many wrote to tell me that it was a great help so I'm going to repeat it here.

Obviously, you can apply the Phonetic Alphabet, but—instead of thinking four, six, nine, two, five (46925) think "four sixty-nine twenty-five" (or "four sixty-nine and a *quarter*"). "Talk" it to yourself (which, when you get right down to it, is what you do when you're thinking). You'll save the back-and-forth to the computer because it will stay with you for those crucial few seconds. That's because instead of thinking five separate entities, you're thinking of only *two*: "four sixty-nine" and "quarter."

For 32650, you can think "three twenty-six fifty" or "three twenty-six and a half." It's a more rhythmic thought (yes, I had to think "*Red Hot You Two-Headed Monster!*"), more fluent and therefore easier to repeat mentally. For 431728, think "four thirty-one seven twenty-eight."

Of course, if you wanted to remember the numbers in the above examples for any length of time, if they were important and you wanted them to become *knowledge,* you'd want to associate what they represented to *reshape nail, munch less, roamed can off.*

Park Here

Do you spend many aggravating minutes searching for your car in a large parking lot or garage? I never do, because I *always* create an image in my mind, as I lock my car, to *tell me* the aisle/location, or whatever. If it's in aisle D2, I visualize my car in my *den* or I connect it to *dean/Noah*. If it's in aisle 4, I'm driving a large bottle of *rye*. If there's no number, say in a shopping mall parking lot, I see what the nearest store is. If it's Banana Republic, I see myself driving a large *banana*. Later, I'll know that my car is parked opposite Banana Republic. These quick associations are done without breaking physical or mental stride; they take no time at all. And even if they did take a bit of time, think of the time you'd be saving by not having to search for your car.

Another example: You want to remember your appointment with Mr. Salzberg at 312 Main Street on the ninth floor. Form your mental reminders: *salt berg* to *mutton* or *mitten* (312) on a main street (or horse's *mane*) and *bee*s are all over it.

Directions

Talking about addresses reminds me of the cliché that men don't like to ask for directions when lost. I don't mind asking for directions at all. I guess the main reason is that I can memorize those directions. And so can you: just Link them.

Make up a standard image for yourself for right and left. I visualize a boxer throwing a *right* cross, or right jab, for *right*, and a red Communist flag for *left*. You can use *yeast* for east and a cowboy hat, or *vest*, for west. You're told to go to the third light—immediately picture *ma*—and make a right turn. See yourself giving your ma a right-cross punch. Go about two miles (you're punching *Noah* and he *smiles*: miles) to a fork in the road (a gigantic fork is smiling) and take the left fork: the gigantic fork waves a red flag (left), and so on. Try it; it will save a lot of aggravation.

Years ago, on the way to a speaking engagement, I stopped to ask for directions at a gas station. They were quite complicated. I remembered them, of course. I did my thing, and I was booked for another appearance at the same place the following week. Driving there seven days later, I saw the same guy pumping gas at the same gas station. I couldn't resist. I drove in, waited until he came to give me gas, and asked, "Was that a *right* turn at the bank?"

I've told you that it doesn't matter if you use a Substitute Word that doesn't sound exactly like the word you want to remember, and that's true. But on rare occasions, it *does matter*. Talking about directions reminded me of the following.

My wife, Renée, and I were visiting the South of France for the first time. It was the summer of 1971. We had rented a villa in Cap-d'Ail, on the Moyenne Corniche, between Nice and Monte Carlo. During our driving explorations in and around Nice, we'd invariably get lost. I used the Nice train station (La Gare) as my "location point." From there, I knew how to drive to our villa. So, when I was lost, I'd ask, *"Pardon, ou est la gare?"* ("Excuse me, where is the train station?").

The problem was that my French was just about nonexistent (I get by pretty well now) and I was pronouncing *gare* to rhyme with "care" instead of the proper way, to rhyme with "ci*gar*." So what I was actually asking was, "Where is the *war*?" (*Ou est la guerre?*).

Most every French person I asked smiled, knew I was American and was simply mispronouncing the word. For a few, I had to say "choo-choo" before they answered, but answer they did. I realized my mistake near the end of that summer, when we were totally lost in the hills of Nice. There was no one in sight except one very old man.

He tottered in our direction. I rolled down my window and said, *"Pardon, monsieur, ou est la gare?"* mispronouncing it "guerre," of course.

The old man stopped, stood staring at me with wide eyes for a moment. Then—and I wish I could show you a photo, it's so clear in my mind—he held out both hands, palms up, as if in supplication, and said with surprise, some concern, and a bit of fear, ending in a "small" question mark: *"C'est fini!?"* (It's finished!?").

I never again asked for the location of the war!

214

Acronyms and More

Earlier in the book I mentioned the use of "every good boy does fine" to remember the lines of a music staff (and *face* to remember the spaces) and the use of HOMES to remember the names of the five Great Lakes. (I used *On Each Hill Man Stands* to remember them in size order.)

This concept occasionally comes in handy. Just about every medical doctor I've ever spoken to has told me that he or she used the following in medical school to help remember the cranial nerves:

On Old Olympia's Towering Top
A Finn and German Vault and Hop.

Of course, they had to know the names of the nerves before the first letters would help remind them of optic, olfactory, oculomotor, trochlear, trigeminal, abducens, facial, auditory, glossopharyngeal, vagus, accessory, and hypoglossal.

The same is true when using SCALP to help remember the layers of the scalp: skin, close connective tissue, aponeurosis (epicranial), loose connective tissue, pericranium.

One medical student told me that he knew the parts of the brain—cerebrum, cerebellum, medulla, oblongata, pons, diencephalon—but needed a way to be reminded of them, to pass his tests. I made up the following silly phrase for him:

Carrying Cargo Makes Old Pants Dirty

It worked. But a quick Link of simple Substitute Word reminders would do as well: *broom* to *bell* to *dull* (or *dollar*) to *long* to *puns* to *save alone.*

Associate STAB to a singing quartet and you'll be reminded that the quartet consists of a soprano, tenor, alto, and bass.

The silly name *Roy B. Giv* reminds me of the colors of the spectrum: red, orange, yellow, blue, green, indigo, violet. It would do the same for you.

Trivia

Oh, so long ago I wanted to remember the names of the seven dwarfs in "Snow White," so I could show off for my little friends. What's interesting here is that I still remember the silly phrase I devised—and I'm talking about seven decades ago! The phrase is: *Double S, Double D and a BiG H.* And that nonsense phrase still reminds me of Sleepy, Sneezy, Doc, Dopey, Bashful, Grumpy, and Happy!

I did the same thing when, for "trivia purposes," I wanted to remember the names of the Dionne quintuplets. You young "whippersnappers" of only fifty or sixty years of age might not know who I'm talking about, but that's okay. It's the idea that's important. I used the acronym MACEY and visualized Macy's department store full of people who looked alike. MACEY, of course, helped me remember Marie, Annette, Cecile, Emily, Yvonne. At this writing, Mary and Cecile are the two surviving sisters, but at the time I'm talking about, only Emily had passed away and that "odd" *e* in the acronym *told* me that.

You see, it really doesn't matter what you use, how silly you get, so long as it comes to you at that time, and *works*. Once I needed to get the digits 0384 in mind quickly: quickly, because other numbers were coming at me rapidly so I had no time to really think. I thought of "some*v*ere," which transposes to 0384.

I'd better explain. When I was a small boy an older man (Mr. Fried) and his dog (Frieda) lived in the same tenement building I did. We used to talk a lot. He spoke with an accent, *v*'s instead of *w*'s, and said the word "somevere" instead of "somewhere" often. Now, at the time the above happened, I didn't think of the word, *samovar,* because I didn't *know* the word, *samovar*. But, and this is the point, I thought of Mr. Fried, and "somevere" automatically came to mind. I hadn't thought of Mr. Fried in many years at the time, but it worked. Just about anything will work for you, if it fits into my "patterns," and if *you* think of it.

Dates

Would you like always to remember that the Great Chicago Fire happened in 1871? Just connect *chick fire* to *cot* (71) or *dove cot* if you think you need to be reminded of the 18. The San Francisco earthquake happened in 1906: connect *sash* or *sage* to earthquake and you'll always know it. Visualize the *Titanic* (*tie tan, hick*) made of *tin* and you'll know that it sank in 19*12*. (See the gigantic tin ship sinking in a gigantic *tub* if you "need" a reminder for 19.)

To remember that Neil Armstrong was the first man to walk on the moon in 1969, think of a muscular (*strong*) *arm* pushing a *ship* (69) to the moon. Here's a way for you to remember *the month* as well as the *year.* Make the first consonant (or first two consonants for November or December) represent the month and the following consonants, the year. Associating *kneel arm strong* to *ketchup* (or *catch up*) would do it because *ketchup*, in this concept, must represent the seventh month (July) of '69.

Here's another way to handle it: Shakespeare was born on April 26, 1564. Imagine you're on a *ranch* (4th month, 26th day) *shak*ing a *spear* in a *tall jar* (1564). To remind yourself of only the month and year, you could use *rattle chair* or *rattle jar* (4-1564).

Abraham Lincoln was assassinated in 1865. See it happening in *jail*, or the perpetrator is tossed into jail.

Does anyone remember the name of Lincoln's first vice president? Think of the last three letters of Lincoln's first name (*ham*) and the first three of his second name (*lin*) and you have the name of Vice President *Hamlin*.

It's nice when things fall into that kind of pattern. For example, as I mentioned much earlier in this book, I'll always know the height of

Mount Fujiyama because, when I was just a schoolboy, I associated it to a calendar. Why a *calendar*? Because there are 12 months in a calendar year and 365 days. Mount Fujiyama is 12,365 feet high. How could I ever forget that? But don't look for things like that, they rarely occur, and it'd take too much time to look for them. If they're obvious then use them, of course.

James Madison was our fourth president. Associate *mad at son* or *medicine* to *rye*. If you want to, get *aims* in the picture to remind you of James. Perhaps you're aiming a spoonful of medicine at a gigantic loaf of rye bread.

The twenty-seventh president was William Taft. *Daft* or *raft* to *neck* will remind you of that. Hayes was the nineteenth president: *hay* or *haze* to *tub* is all you need. You can learn all the presidents this way. Again, what a good mental exercise that'd be.

Do It Now

I'll give you one more "rule" that will certainly improve your memory. It's a cliché rule, but one that surely works. The rule is *DO IT NOW*. My sub-rule is, try not to let a paper go through your hands more than once. Because if you do, what too often happens is, you drop the paper somewhere on your desk with the thought, "I'll take care of it later." It gets covered up with other papers and you never see it again! It's forgotten. Take care of it *now*; then you can't forget it.

And even if you don't forget it, you'll spend valuable time searching for it. A Harvard Business School study reveals that the average executive (no matter how old) wastes about thirty minutes a day searching for papers on his or her desk. That's lots of hours per year. Do it *now* and that search is no longer necessary. "I'll do it later" is procrastination, not only at the office but at home. "Oh, I'll call so-and-so later" is almost like not calling at all, or calling too late.

I'm not suggesting that you can *always* "do it now," but you can surely do it now much more often than you're doing it now!

Here and There

I realize that I've jumped around a bit in this chapter—because I wanted to touch on a variety of ideas that, if they interest you, can be enlarged upon. Since there's no way I can touch on *every* strategy, *every* memory problem, I wanted to give you some ideas to work on yourself.

For example, do you miss the "good old days" when you could simply walk up to the counter of your local drugstore, ask for your razor blades or face cream, and get the product immediately, pay, and leave? Nowadays, drugstores take up thousands of square feet of space and you have to search for your items (unless you are lucky enough to find someone to ask).

Well, I visualize a gigantic *bee* shaving to tell me that shaving stuff is in aisle 9 in my drugstore. A sheet of *tin* (or a tin can) is shampooing: shampoos are in aisle 12. A judge (*law*) is banging on the bench with a gigantic bottle of aspirin (the pills fly all over the place): aspirin is in aisle 5.

The same applies to your supermarket. Once I picture my *toes* sticking together because there is honey all over them, how can I *not* know that honey is in aisle 10? Coffee is in aisle 2, so I "see" cans of coffee marching onto the ark (*Noah*—2) two by two. Save yourself time, effort, and aggravation. Simply apply my techniques.

I never dogear the pages of a book I'm reading. When I want to stop and go to sleep, I see the book (for example) being *tired.* The next time I pick up that book, I automatically turn to page 141! If I had visualized a gigantic book at the stove, making an *omelette,* I'd know that I had stopped reading on page 351. No bookmarks or dogears necessary.

SRETTEL

Here's a silly mental exercise for you. People are always asking me if I can recite the alphabet backward. (Link your alphabet words from *zebra* to *ape* and you *can*.) I have gone a step further, which is my wont. I write this on paper or blackboard, rapidly:

ZAYBXCWDVEUFTGSHRIQJPKOLNM

It's the alphabet *forward and backward at the same time*! Start at the left and move to the right, skipping every other letter; then, at the N, go left, again skipping every other letter. All I did, many years ago, was to set up these reminders: *Say bee* (ZAYB), *eggs see water* (XCW), *the view* (DVEU), *foot gasher* (FTGSHR), *IQ* of a *Jeep* (IQJP), *call name* (KOLNM).

Try to visualize the reminders. You might see yourself talking to a bee, saying, "Say, bee." After you go over them a few times, this will remind you of ZAYB. You're pointing at *eggs*, asking if they *see w*ater (I just think "eggs, see W?" for XCW), also see the view (DVEU). As you talk, someone gashes your foot, he's a foot gasher (FTGSHR); tell him that he has the IQ of a Jeep (IQJP); he calls you a name (KOLNM).

Well, you said you wanted a silly mental exercise; it sure is more fun than doing a crossword puzzle.

SPECIAL MIND-POWER EXERCISE #29

$2 + 11 - 1 = 12$

The above is a correct equation. Can you prove that it's correct with *letters* of the alphabet instead of numbers?

This is unique. I know of no other equation that *can* be "shown" with letters in this way.

Think about it, exercise your mind.

So, we've reached the end of our time together. It's been fun for me and, I hope, for you. I also hope that you've tried to apply all of the ideas I've tried to implant, and that you're not waiting until you get a *Round Tuitt*.

That is, you're not reading, agreeing, nodding, and thinking, "Wow, I'll learn this and try it when I get *around to it*." Boy, I sure wish I could manufacture "Round Tuitts": I'd sell millions of them. No, don't wait. Learn and apply my systems now. Build more brain cells. Keep your mind young for the rest of your life. The fact to bear in mind is that you have absolutely nothing to lose. What if my systems don't work and you forget things? So what? What's changed? You've been doing *that* for years! You'll still be giving your mind a needed and important workout. No, you have nothing to lose, but so much to gain.

Quite a few years ago, as noted in *Health Magazine*, research at the Albert Einstein College of Medicine found that stimulating the mind "actually causes rewiring of the brain, the sprouting of new synapses." This was told to the *Washington Post* by Joseph Coyle of Harvard University. He went on to say that "exercising the mind offers powerful protection against mental deterioration." So you see, I haven't been lying to you!

Stop waiting until you get a Round Tuitt. The bit of effort needed to apply the skills I've taught in this book is quite painless. Sure, a bit of effort is necessary. What worthwhile thing is ever accomplished without a bit of effort? All you need to do is—*do it*! If you are concerned about the effort involved in applying the systems, stop and think of the effort and work involved when you had to apply *rote* memory, which rarely works well, if at all.

I've said it before and it's important enough for me to say it again: my memory-training technique is the only art or skill I know of that you can start applying *now*, immediately. Applying it is your practice and, before you know it, applying my systems, tricks, and strategies will be automatic—and won't involve expending much effort at all.

Out of every thousand students I might come across perhaps two "Yeah buts" or "What ifs." They're the kind of people who rarely learn anything new because they're busy "Yeah butting" and "What iffing" instead of applying and doing. They're typical of those who wait for a Round Tuitt. Don't, please don't, fall into that category. The systems taught here have been proven for more years than I care to remember(!). Just start applying them and your "Yeah buts" or "What ifs" will simply fade away, they'll be answered automatically as you proceed and progress.

Once, I was teaching how to remember foreign language vocabulary using ten words to start. Everyone applied my system and knew the words after hearing them only once. Then one student "Yeah butted" me: "Yeah, but there are thousands of words to remember when learning a foreign language." My answer: "So? Don't you see that if there were only ten or twenty words in a language you wouldn't need my techniques? It's when there *are* thousands that you *need* my systems, that's when they 'shine'!" It's so obvious, isn't it?

The cliché is that we use about 10 percent of our mental capacities. I believe that that's giving most people the benefit of the doubt! In any case, learn and apply what I've taught you here, do the Mind-Power Exercises, and you'll be using much more of your mental capacity than most. (You really began doing just that starting with the third chapter of this book!)

Listen—knowledge is acquired in only one way. New information is attached to, connected to, *associated* with, what we *already* know. We start out knowing very little: you couldn't read until that "knowledge" was connected to what you already knew, the letters and the sounds the letters make.

It's an upside-down pyramid. New knowledge is attached to that narrow bottom point and that narrow point starts to expand upward and outward, creating that upside-down pyramid. The *older* we get, the wiser we get, the more knowledge we accrue, the taller and wider grows that pyramid. That's how I've been teaching you. I taught you how to make one thing consciously remind you of another. Then I taught you how to form Substitute Words or

Thoughts to make abstract information tangible in your mind. I taught you how to "see" names, numbers, words, and so much more; I've built a "pyramid" of knowledge for you in this, my area of expertise.

I've been told that if I could "bottle" my systems, it'd be a boon to society. Well, I've come as close to that as I could, I've "bottled" them here in this book. Now, it's your turn to do *something:* you have to *uncork that bottle!*

Stop waiting to get a Round Tuitt. Here's the simple, easy-to-apply rule for learning anything new. It's a basic one-word rule derived from the two-word rule, "do it." Here it is:

BEGIN.

SOLUTIONS TO THE SPECIAL MIND-POWER EXERCISES

Exercise #1

Some of your friends will "see" this right away (as you may have), others will take some time to solve it (as you may have). Those who stay only in the Roman numeral "rut" are the ones who will have trouble with it.

I never said that the even number had to be a Roman numeral. If you thought outside the usual boundaries—that is, exercised your mind—you saw that the symbol to place in front of the IX is the letter S. That changes *IX* to the word for the even number *SIX*.

One of my goals is to help you get out of that "thinking rut" in which most of us spend our lives.

Exercise #2

I'm afraid this one is a bit of a "groaner." The riddle *tells* you the answer.

> Forward I'm heavy, *backward I'm NOT*.
> The answer is the word *TON*. Backward, that word is *NOT*.

Exercise #3

The wise old Arab simply adds his own camel to the 17, bringing the total number of camels to 18. Then, the camels are divided as follows:

> 1/2 of 18 is 9 camels for number one son.
> 1/3 of 18 is 6 camels for number two son.
> 1/9 of 18 is 2 camels for number three son.

After each son takes his allotted camels (9 + 6 + 2 = *17*), the wise old Arab's camel remains. He mounts it and rides off into the sandstorm.

Exercise #4

There's an excellent trap or "throw-off" built into this seemingly easy-to-solve exercise. That's why it's rare that anyone gets it right the first (or sometimes second or third) time.

Most people answer *eleven*. That's because they mentally go through the numbers 1 to 99, thinking, "6, 16, 26, 36, 46, 56…Ah ha! *There's* the catch: 66. *Two* sixes there. He won't fool me with *that*."

So, they count two sixes for 66 and continue, "76, 86, 96," arriving at *eleven* sixes.

The 66 is actually a "red herring" that makes you overlook the real "catch": 60, 61, 62, 63, 64, 65, 66, 67, 68, 69!

The correct answer is: The painter will have painted *twenty* sixes.

Exercise #5

Here's what you do: Throw switch 1 to "on." Leave it at "on" for a few minutes.

Then switch 1 to "off" and throw switch 2 to "on."

Immediately walk to the room where the lightbulb is. If the light is on, there's no problem, you know that 2 is the "real" switch.

But if the bulb isn't on…*feel* the bulb. (That's why I told you that the bare bulb was hanging low.) If it feels warm, then 1 is the "real" switch. If it's cold, then the real switch must be 3.

The switch numbers I have given here are just examples. You can use whichever you like. Going in order, though—1, 2, 3—is probably the easiest way to work it.

Exercise #6

This is one of those problems that makes you think, "Oh, of course!" the instant you see the answer.

The letters are NOTABLE.

The NOTABLE surgeon was NOT ABLE to operate because he had NO TABLE.

Exercise #7

Once you see the concept behind this one, it's easy to solve.

Mrs. Johnson starts with fifteen oranges.

She gives the first friend exactly half of them (seven and a half) plus half an orange—that's seven and a half plus one half, or eight. She's left with seven oranges.

The second friend gets half of seven (three and a half) oranges, plus half an orange—or four. Mrs. Johnson is left with three oranges.

The third friend gets half of three (one and a half) plus half an orange—two.

This leaves Mrs. Johnson with one orange.

You can make it slightly easier by having Mrs. J bump into only two friends. Same problem, same wording, same ending—and same reasoning, except that Mrs. J starts with *seven* oranges.

Exercise #8

Fill the five-gallon bucket, then pour the contents out of it into the three-gallon bucket.

When the three-gallon bucket is full, there are two gallons left in the five-gallon bucket.

Empty and discard the contents of the three-gallon bucket, then pour the two gallons of water in the five-gallon bucket into the three-gallon bucket. You've now isolated exactly two gallons of water in the three-gallon bucket.

Simply fill the five-gallon bucket from the water hose and you have five gallons in it, and two gallons in the other bucket: *seven* gallons.

Exercise #9

An English teacher is discussing a student's essay with another teacher and she says: *"That 'that' that that boy used is absolutely correct."*

Exercise #10

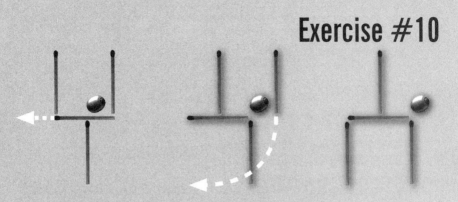

You really do move only two matches, but one moves rather strangely—only halfway, like this: Slide the only horizontal match, the bottom of the "glass," just above the stem, *halfway* to the left, as in the first illustration.

Then move the match at the right, the one near the olive, to the left and down, to form the left side of the upsidedown glass. The end result is exactly the same glass, but upside down with the olive outside, as in the third illustration.

Simple, when you know how!

Exercise #11

I never said that you had to stay *within* the square formed by the nine dots. If you locked yourself into that thinking rut, you couldn't solve this. If, however, you exercised your mind a bit more and thought, "Hey, I can make some lines *outside* the square," you may have solved it—because that is the way to arrive at the solution:

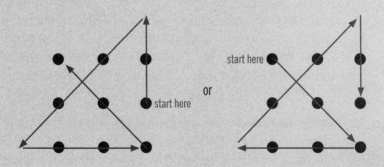

Exercise #12

The first thing you have to do is label the bags 1, 2, 3, 4, and 5.

Then take one coin out of bag 1, two coins out of bag 2, three coins out of 3, four coins out of 4, and five coins out of 5.

If all the coins were legitimate, the five bags together (15 ounces each) would weigh 75 ounces. Removing 15 coins as explained removes 15 ounces. So, the fifteen bags should now weigh exactly 60 ounces.

Now all you have to do is weigh all five bags together, once. The number of grams you're short *tells* you which is the bag with the counterfeit coins. If the scale shows that you're *three* grams short, then bag 3 contains the counterfeit coins, etc.

Exercise #13

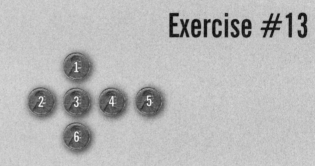

Pick up coin 5 and place it *onto* coin 3. You've moved only one coin and now there are four coins in the horizontal row and four coins in the vertical row.

Exercise #14

The answer is *one*.

The key is that you *know* all three boxes are incorrectly labeled. So, remove one marble from the box labeled **BW** (black/white) and follow along:

Assume that the marble you remove is black. Then you also know for a fact that the other marble in that box is also black. Why? Because if it was white, then the box would be *correctly* labeled (**BW**), and you know that's not so. Slap the **BB** label on that box.

Once you know you have the correct label on one box, the rest is easy. Remove the **WW** label from its box and replace it with the **BW** label. (You *know* that **WW** is incorrect. And it can't contain two blacks because you've just identified the "real" **BB** box with the **BB** label. So it *must* be **BW**.)

The remaining box can only be the one that holds the two white marbles. The **WW** label goes on that.

(Another way to look at it is this: after you've properly placed the **BB** label, you're holding the **BW** label in your hand. Switch it with the **WW** label and tack the one in your hand *now* [**WW**] onto the one remaining box.)

The same reasoning applies if the one marble you take out of the **BW** box is white. Slap the **WW** label on that box; switch the in-hand **BW** label with the **BB** label and stick the one now in your hand (**BB**) onto the remaining unlabeled box.

Another way to present this great mind exercise is to tell your friend that it can be done by removing only one marble. He or she has to figure out *how*.

Exercise #15

Your mental exercise was to think of one word to which you could add just one syllable and make it shorter.

The answer, of course, is *short*. Add the syllable "er" to *short* and you have *shorter*.

Exercise #16

I told you that there were two hints in the way I worded the problem. I purposely used the words "strong" and "length" to make you subconsciously think of the eight-letter, one-vowel word **STRENGTH**.

Another "word" kind of thinking exercise is to think of a common English word that contains all five vowels in their proper sequence. It's a good conversation starter or ice-breaker. That word is *facetious*.

Exercise #17

What I'm purchasing (probably in a hardware store) are those numbers that you glue onto your outside mailbox or door to show your address.

> Each number sticker or patch costs ten cents. So, the 1 is ten cents.
>
> 43 costs twenty cents because you need the 4 patch and the 3 patch.
>
> 123 costs thirty cents because you need three patches—and so on.

Exercise #18

Here are the five single odd digits placed so that they add up to an even number.

$$\begin{array}{r} 1\,1 \\ 1 \\ 1 \\ \underline{1} \\ 14 \end{array}$$

Exercise #19

To purchase exactly 100 birds and spend exactly $100, you need to buy:

94 chickens at 50 cents each	$ 47
1 duck at $3 each	$ 3
5 turkeys at $10 each	$ 50
	$100

Exercise #20

Five cards can be laid out in 120 different ways.

> The way to reach that conclusion is to multiply 5 x 4 x 3 x 2 x 1 = 120.

Four items: 4 x 3 x 2 x 1 = 24

Six items can be laid out in 720 ways. Check it out.

The "extra little mind exercise" at the end of chapter 20

There are six F's in that paragraph. Most people tend to overlook the "of"s. Read it again and see.

Exercise #21

In all of "numberdom," the only number that tells you how many letters it is spelled with is:

FOUR
(It's spelled with *four* letters.)

Exercise #22

Assume the digits below are your ten coins:

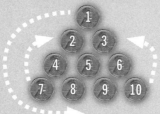

Move 7 and 10 up to the left/right of 2 and 3. Then move 1 down to under and between 8 and 9. Now the arrow points downward.

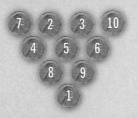

Exercise #23

The solution may seem more complicated than the problem itself—so you'll get a bit more mental exercise. The key is to make it *immaterial* whether it's a T or an L person standing at the fork in the road. And that's done by *pointing* to either road, and asking:

"If I had asked you *before* would you have said that this is the road to Kumbawa?"

It's the past-tense concept that does it. If you're pointing to the correct road as you ask this question of either a T or an L person, the answer must be "yes." If you're indicating the wrong road as you ask it, either type of person would have to say "no."

Assume you're pointing to the correct road. A T person would have said yes before (remember, he always tells the truth), therefore his answer now is also yes.

An L person, who always lies, would have lied before, and said no. You're asking him if he *would have* said it's the correct road. Well, he wouldn't have, he'd have lied and said no. Since he has to lie now, for this current question, he does lie, and says yes.

That reasoning also applies if you're pointing to the wrong road and asking the same question. The T person will have to say no; the L person must also say no.

I'm hoping I've explained this clearly so that you can follow it, otherwise you're going to get lost on your way to Kumbawa!

Exercise #24

Look at the first illustration; that's what you'll have to remember if you want to do my "instant" magic square.

You can use the Phonetic Alphabet to help you do so. You need to be able to think, without hesitation,

"8,11,14,1   13,2,7,12   3,16,9,6   10,5,4,15"

When you're given a number for your square, fill in twelve of those numbers—but different numbers, according to the total you want, go into the blanks shown in the second illustration.

8	11	14	1
13	2	7	12
3	16	9	6
10	5	4	15

8	11		1
	2	7	12
3		9	6
10	5	4	

You've drawn your blank 4 x 4 square. Now assume you're given the number 64. You can instantly start filling in 8, 11 and **subtract 20** (always) from the given number (64, this example) to put into the original 14 square; 44 goes there, and the 1 goes into the upper-right square. Write **one less** than the 44 (this example) in the next (original 13) square so 43 goes there. Do the 2, 7, 12. Then, the next row—3—and write the number that's **two higher** than the 44 you put in the top row; so 46 goes into that empty third row square.

Do 9, 6. Then do the 10, 5, 4 and write **one higher** than the 44 in that last square— 45 goes there. And you've completed the magic square for 64. Check it.

This will work exactly this way for **any** number over 34. It's easier to fill in the last square in the last row with 45, then jump to the third row to write the 46. There's less "thinking" necessary that way. Just go over the examples; it will all lock in for you soon enough. Then go back to the exercise to refresh your memory as to all the patterns that add to the selected number.

8	11	44	1
43	2	7	12
3	46	9	6
10	5	4	45

You're really exercising your mind now!

Exercise #25

Actually, the hint—that these are prices I found in a 7-Eleven store—is the answer!

If you add the four prices—$3.16, $1.20, $1.25, $1.50—you'll see that they add to $7.11.

What's unique about them is that if you *multiply* them, the answer is also $7.11!

$3.16 \times 1.20 \times 1.25 \times 1.50 = 7.11$

Exercise #26

The coins in your pocket or purse that total $1.19 are four pennies, four dimes, one quarter, and one half dollar.

With those coins you can't make change for a dollar, half dollar, quarter, dime, or nickel.

Exercise #27

Remove one book from the balancing scale's left side, leaving two books there. Then remove the one book from the scale's right side, leaving only the half-pound weight.

You now have two books on the left and only the half-pound weight on the right, and the scale is perfectly balanced.

Since the two books weigh exactly the same as the half-pound weight, and you know that all the books weigh the same amount, then each book must weigh a quarter of a pound.

Exercise #28

The hint I gave you was, "it's worth a drink." The common six-letter word is

BRANDY

You were told to remove one letter at a time until you couldn't remove any more letters. That should have told you that you'd have to end with a one-letter word. There are only two of those in English: *I* and *a.* Here's the whole solution:

BRANDY

BRAND

BRAN

RAN

AN

A

Exercise #29

$$2 + 11 - 1 = 12$$

Watch:

TWO + ELEVEN, or TWOELEVEN, represents $2 + 11$.

For the "minus 1" *take away* O N E by crossing out those letters, like this:

TW̶O̶EL̶E̶VEN̶

to leave TWELVE!

INDEX